How to do a Systematic Literature Review in Nursing

A Step-by-Step Guide

3rd edition

How to do a Systematic Literature Review in Nursing

A Step-by-Step Guide

3rd edition

Josette Bettany-Saltikov and Robert McSherry

 Open University Press

Open University Press
McGraw Hill
Unit 4
Foundation Park
Roxborough Way
Maidenhead
SL6 3UD

email: emea_uk_ireland@mheducation.com
world wide web: www.mheducation.co.uk

First published 2012
Second edition published 2016
First published in this third edition 2024

Executive Editor: Sam Crowe
Editorial Assistant: Hannah Jones
Content Product Manager: Graham Jones

A catalogue record of this book is available from the British Library

ISBN-13: 9780335251148
ISBN-10: 0335251145
eISBN-13: 9780335251155

Typeset by Transforma Pvt. Ltd., Chennai, India
Printed and bound by CPI Group (UK) Ltd, Croydon, CR0 4YY

Praise page

Now in its third edition, Bettany-Saltikov and McSherry's textbook provides a comprehensively updated version of their internationally popular step-by-step guide to conducting a systematic literature review in nursing. Taking us through each phase, in an easy-to-read format, Bettany-Saltikov and McSherry once again provide the reader with a road map that easily enables the conduct of the review. Essential elements such as developing a focused research question and specifying objectives, place the scholar in a good position to move forward on a manageable and robust systematic review. These authors clearly outline further steps necessary for success, including the skills of systematic searching, methods of critical appraisal and synthesizing and writing up the review. The book is very engaging for the reader. Practical tips are interspersed throughout the book that permit the reader to draw essential easy to remember material from each chapter. The authors also provide a comprehensive range of templates that are very useful to support the work required for the review process. Summaries, key points, and short reflective questions at end of chapters allow readers to quickly absorb and remember important information from each chapter. These also serve as a quick go to reminder. While the book provides a comprehensive guide to the process of systematic review, each chapter also stands alone as an important resource for each sub element of the process, that can be easily understood independently. Overall, this book provides a solid basis for nurses embarking on the systematic review and provides information and resources that enable clear understanding and ultimately success in what can be a challenging process. Fundamentally the book empowers nurses to embrace the skills necessary to embark upon evidence-based practice, an essential element that ensures continued excellence and advancement in healthcare."

Fiona Timmins PhD, FAAN, MSc, BNS, BSc Health and Social Care (Open) BA (Open), FFNRCSI, RGN; Professor of Nursing, Dean, and Head of School at the School of Nursing, Midwifery and Health Systems, University College Dublin, Ireland and Editor in Chief of Public Health Nursing Journal.

"Working with vulnerable service users and patients it is essential that your practice is current and underpinned by the evidence. This is a requirement not only of nurses but of all professional bodies. Nurses, health care professionals and their students need to be able to understand and interpret current research articles.

This book is a comprehensive resource to explain the what, when, why, and how to complete a systematic literature review. It is invaluable book for all nurses and health care professionals who want to be able to interpret research in order to deliver evidence based practice to the people they work with."

Margaret Spencer, Consultant Occupational Therapist OT360, UK

"Whoever you are, and whatever your background, if you want to know what makes a good systematic review, then get a copy of this third edition by Bettany-Saltikov and McSherry. In this era, where there is a tsunami of evidence and conflicting views about research, clear authoritative guidance on how to carry out robust systematic reviews is more important than ever. Quality always pays off in the end, so treat yourself to a copy of this book which explains all you need to know about systematic reviews with a step-by-step guide in language that is easy to understand."

Dr Ray Samuriwo, Associate Professor in Nursing, School of Health and Social Care, Edinburgh Napier University, UK

"This third edition of this highly essential book continues to provide nurses at pre and post -registration level with the step-by-step essential information of 'how to' undertake a systematic review of existing literature. The ability to systematically search, appraise and answer research questions from existing literature is fundamental in nursing where nurses must always be evidence informed in their practice. The authors have managed to ensure the language of research is penetrable and the helpful way chapters create the step-by step approach to conducting a review from creation of a question to how to synthesise findings will develop confidence in the nurse. Although aimed at those undertaking a systematic review this book will also be an essential read for any supervisor supporting students and I will be utilising this with my students".

Dr Nicola Clarke, Associate Professor of Reflective Academic Practice, Birmingham City University, UK

"'Step by step' is exactly what senior undergraduate students undertaking their research /dissertation modules require. This text fulfils its promise. It has a logical and clear structure. It guides the reader through all stages of the process, using uncomplicated language, thus demystifying what can be a daunting task for many students.

The inclusion of 'practical tip' and 'key points' boxes encourage the reader to review their understanding of the chapter content. The 'Q&A' boxes are very useful and cover many of the questions raised by students undertaking this task for the first time. Chapters contain useful templates and diagrammatic explanations where possible, this will be helpful for students with all types of learning styles. The inclusion of examples from students' actual dissertations provides the encouragement that 'you can do this too'. The case studies are useful when trying to understand the research process from a clinical perspective.

Students from other health professions, should be able to appreciate the links to practice being made, despite the inclusion of mainly nursing examples. The text could have easily been written for students of all health professions in mind, maybe worthy of another version (different title) of the same content, with less nursing focused examples included?

This text should be a 'go to' for students from any health care profession, just because it has 'nursing' in its title – it should not be overlooked. This text is an asset to help any healthcare student successfully complete their undergraduate degree."

Amanda Blaber, RGN, BSc(Hons), MSc, PGCE, Advance HE; Honorary Fellow College of Paramedics; Freelance Writer; Retired Senior Lecturer with over 20 years' experience teaching nursing and paramedic students in several Higher Education Institutions.

"This guidebook could be hand-written for qualified nurses wishing to enhance their approach to evidence-based nursing, or nursing students studying at all academic levels. It's strengths rest within its logical structure based on clearly defined chapters, which relate to each stage of the systematic literature review process. The book provides practical tips and hyperlinks to key websites and organisations. Each process is clearly illustrated through diagrams, tables and case studies, and templates are helpfully included. It is written in an encouraging, relatable style which will give readers a sense of confidence and facilitate rigorous practice."

Dr Warren Stewart, RN, Ed D, MA, BSc (Hons), School of Education, Sport and Health Sciences, University of Brighton, UK

"This 3rd edition of How to do a Systematic Literature Review in Nursing by Bettany-Saltikov and McSherry is a practical and accessible textbook, for nursing students or those already qualified. It is a useful resource which offers comprehensive definitions and detailed step by step instructions to guide the reader in understanding of how undertake a systematic review. It is further aided by examples of real nursing practice issues, which are translated into research questions and developed into illustrative examples throughout the textbook. Each chapter has a specific focus on an element of the systematic review process, which

provides templates, completed examples, key learning points, hints, tips, followed by a summary and questions and answers. This updated version includes a new chapter which introduces meta-analysis. Overall, this textbook is a great companion for anyone wanting to learn more about research principles and how to undertake a systematic review."

Angelina Chadwick, Lecturer in Mental Health Nursing, University of Salford, UK

Contents

List of boxes

List of figures

List of tables

Foreword

The demand for nursing and healthcare practice to be evidence based is driven by societal expectations and improved technologies for the production, dissemination, searching and access of published research. We are fortunate to live in an age where research-driven healthcare is the standard. However, the potential for information overload, and the difficulty of assessing the credibility of the evidence, has led to a greater demand by practitioners for an unbiased synthesis of the evidence.

Today's nurses and health professionals need the skills and knowledge to find, evaluate and amalgamate evidence to use in practice. Editors must be assured that their published literature reviews are credible and safe. The wider society needs to trust that nursing and healthcare practitioners are giving them the best care, according to the evidence. Although nursing and healthcare practice is a combination of ethics, empathetic care, practical skills, critical thinking and knowledge – all combined in the moment of action in the world – there is no doubt that understanding and applying evidence within their role is a fundamental requirement of nurses and healthcare professionals' registration and role.

This book has many excellent qualities that make it essential reading for undergraduate and practising nurses and healthcare professionals:

- It clearly outlines the relationship between systematically reviewing the evidence and professional practice.
- It uses accessible language but, by explaining the reasons for each aspect of the literature review from first principles, it takes the aspiring reviewer from beginner to expert.
- In addition to the step-by-step guide that explains the process of undertaking a systematic literature review, it also provides document outlines and tools for the reader to use in carrying out their own systematic review.
- It provides links to many useful resources that can be used to enhance knowledge and the quality of a systematic review.
- It uses accessible examples of literature search questions and strategies that make it easier for readers to develop their own review.

If nursing research is to develop and become embedded within practice, then we all need to know how to use it, how to synthesize what is known in order to take the next step in discovery, and how to explain and apply it for our colleagues to use. The authors explain what we owe to Archie Cochrane in his demand for evidence-based practice in medicine. In a similar vein, I have used the previous editions of this textbook for teaching students how to carry out systematic reviews, and to guide my own work, over many years. Nurses have learned how to synthesize evidence for presentation to colleagues, to inform policy and to develop their own research questions by using this textbook. This updated edition provides the tools for us to continue growing the conceptual bases for nursing and applying them to practice for the benefit of all.

Dr Hazel M Chapman
Postgraduate tutor/senior lecturer
University of Chester, Faculty of Health, Medicine and Society
8 March 2024

Acknowledgements

It is with great pleasure and gratitude that we present this third edition. In the years following the publication of the last edition, we have been humbled by the ongoing feedback that we have received regarding the usefulness and value of the book. The primary reason for its popularity, we believe, is the way the book takes the reader through the various steps to complete a systematic review, along with its simplistic and jargon-free style of writing.

Again, we would like to thank our students for kindly giving us permission to use extracts from their dissertations, to allow us to illustrate by example through the case studies within the book. We would also like to thank our undergraduate and postgraduate students for their continued words of encouragement regarding the writing of this third edition. We have learnt as much from you as we hope you have from us. We would also like to thank Kay Caldwell, Lynne Henshaw and Georgina Taylor for kindly permitting us to use their framework in Chapters 8 and 10 of this book. We thank our colleagues, particularly Dr John Franklin for writing the new chapter, 'An introduction to meta-analysis', which was a recommendation by the reviewers. Finally, a BIG THANK YOU to the publishing team for commissioning this edition and for their ongoing support and encouragement throughout the journey of this third edition.

Introduction

We are delighted to introduce this third edition of *How to Do a Systematic Literature Review in Nursing: A Step-by-Step Guide*. We hope you find the third edition as useful and practical as the first and second. The revisions and enhancements to this edition are based on individual and reviewer feedback and published reviews. We also had the second edition sent for independent peer review to several leads for research within academic institutions across the UK. We would like to personally thank these reviewers and all individuals who have so kindly taken the time to provide feedback to help us reshape this third edition.

Since the first publication of the book, we have noticed that the popularity of undertaking a systematic review within undergraduate and postgraduate nursing and allied health professions educational programmes continues to grow. Systematic reviews continue to form part of undergraduate and postgraduate dissertations, fulfilling assessment criteria for research and evidence-based nursing modules, and are taught in final dissertation modules to fulfill the requirements of master's and doctoral degrees. Perhaps the reasons for this are issues associated with achieving ethical approval and/or undertaking live research in a relatively short, fixed period of time – or simply a desire to answer a burning clinical question from practice.

You will notice we have updated the book to provide an even more step-by-step guide, by increasing the content in most chapters and including a new Chapter 13 titled 'An introduction to meta-analysis'. We have done this to help simplify some of the existing information into more 'bite-sized chunks'. We have also retained the case studies, practical tips, questions and answers, and 'key points' sections – all aiming to enhance the progression and quality of your systematic review. We have also included templates to enable you to undertake each part of the systematic literature review process with confidence.

The aim of the book is to continue to provide a simple and practical step-by-step approach to conducting a systematic literature review. We have tried as much as possible to present all the content in this book in a simple and clear format in order to make it suitable for your own abilities, level of learning and available time. This book is intended for all nurses in practice, nursing students, nurse lecturers teaching at universities and other healthcare professionals in a diverse range of settings.

A conversational style has purposely been retained, because several reviews indicated that this was a key strength of the first and second editions and that it was successful in engaging the reader as much as possible. We would like to encourage and not discourage you to see the value of undertaking a systematic review and how this may continue to lead to improvements in patient safety, quality, compassionate care and services in the future. We know from our own and our students' experiences and from undertaking research surrounding evidence-informed nursing that some nurses and student nurses are put off research and research methods if the content that is presented is very academic and full of jargon. We are of the opinion that a systematic literature review (or systematic review) is not only for doctors or high-level Cochrane review researchers. We have found, over the past several years, that anyone with basic undergraduate research skills is able to do this type of review. We can say this confidently because we have taught this method of reviewing to nurses, nursing students and other healthcare professionals over many years.

When we teach systematic literature reviews and the term 'systematic review' is mentioned, many students start panicking and saying, 'I don't know how to do this!' But our combined experience of having taught over one thousand students on a number of dissertation modules has proved that once the individual steps are shown to learners in a straightforward manner, all levels of students – including undergraduate nurses, master's and doctoral students, returning nurses, nurse specialists and practitioners – are indeed able and capable of undertaking a systematic review to completion and to a high standard. Some students have even published their systematic literature reviews. This third edition offers a practical guide to support you step by step, from start to finish of your own systematic literature review. We hope you enjoy this third edition of the book and that you are successful in undertaking your systematic review. The following is a brief overview of the contents of the book:

Chapter 1: What is a systematic review?

This chapter opens by positioning the importance of systematic reviews within the context of evidence-based nursing and the professional nurse cycle. We illustrate how undertaking a systematic review has evolved over time, along with the definitions. We offer our own definition in moving the subject forward for the future. The different types of systematic reviews and common databases for finding these reviews are discussed. We also highlight the differences between literature (narrative) reviews and systematic ones and then debate the hierarchy of evidence.

Chapter 2: Asking an answerable and focused systematic review question

In this chapter the key points to remember when selecting a review topic are described and different ways of narrowing the review topic to a specific question are presented. This is followed by a discussion of the meaning and functions of an answerable and focused review question. The main types of focused research questions are then discussed and some examples from nursing practice are provided. This is followed by a presentation on the different types of research questions and the importance of selecting the appropriate research design for the type of research question you have selected. A number of templates are also provided to help you formulate your own answerable and focused review question.

Chapter 3: Creating the protocol for your systematic review

This chapter highlights the importance of writing a protocol for your review, the steps to take and sections to be included within your protocol. The importance of managing and planning your time is highlighted.

Chapter 4: Writing the background to your systematic review

This chapter details the background information required to prepare your protocol, which will provide an operational definition of the clinical problem. The importance of the review question and grabbing the attention of the reader is highlighted. Issues associated with clarifying the gap in systematic reviews in the clinical area are discussed, as is how to apply different tools and methods to help you start writing up your background section.

Chapter 5: Specifying your objectives and inclusion and exclusion criteria

This chapter discusses the meanings of and differences between a problem statement, an aim, an objective and a review question. Methods for specifying the inclusion and exclusion criteria are discussed and examples provided for different quantitative and qualitative review questions. Templates are also provided to help you write out your own problem statement, aims and objectives as well as your inclusion and exclusion criteria.

Chapter 6: Conducting a comprehensive and systematic literature search

This chapter discusses the importance of undertaking a comprehensive and systematic search, as well as the rationale and aims. The key factors to be considered when undertaking a comprehensive search are described as well as the steps involved in converting your review question into a comprehensive search strategy.

Chapter 7: Working with your primary papers: Stage 1 – Selecting the studies to include in your own systematic review

This chapter discusses working with your primary papers. Stage 1 of this process is associated with selecting the appropriate papers to answer your review question and the methods of the review. The templates to select the papers for your own systematic literature review are detailed.

Chapter 8: Working with your primary papers: Stage 2 – Appraising the methodological quality of your included primary papers

The chapter details Stage 2 of working with your primary papers, which involves appraising the methodological quality of the research studies you have included. We provide the methods of the review, explain how to appraise the methodological quality of the research papers that you have selected and give a worked example of using the framework by Kay Caldwell, Lynne Henshaw and Georgina Taylor to critique a nursing paper.

Chapter 9: Working with your primary papers: Stage 3 – Extracting the data from your included papers

The chapter details the final stage of working with your primary papers, which is associated with extracting data from the papers. The methods of review and how to extract the appropriate data from your included research papers are discussed.

Chapter 10: Synthesizing, summarizing and presenting your findings

This chapter discusses issues to consider when synthesizing and summarizing your results. The tools to use when summarizing and synthesizing your results are offered and ways of how and where to get started on presenting your results are detailed. The chapter includes ways of presenting the results of your search, the results of the studies selected based on the title and abstract, the results of the studies selected based on reading the full paper, a summary of all your included studies, a summary of all the critiques of your included papers using the appropriate frameworks, and summary of the data extracted (including a synthesis of the overall results). We discuss summarizing, synthesizing and presenting your interventions and comparative interventions, outcomes and quantitative and qualitative outcome measures.

Chapter 11: Writing up your discussion and completing your systematic review

This chapter discusses ways of structuring the discussion section of your systematic literature review. Extracts from case studies as well as a completed systematic review are presented and debated. Suggestions for writing up your review report are also described, as are tips for improving academic writing skills.

Chapter 12: Checking your systematic review is complete and a few practical ways to share and disseminate your findings

This chapter provides a systematic review checklist with explanations and the preferred reporting items for systematic reviews and meta-analysis (PRISMA) statements. We also discuss some practical ways to help support you in sharing and disseminating your systematic literature review.

Chapter 13: An introduction to meta-analysis

The final chapter aims to support you in moving towards more advanced methods of data extraction and synthesis. It provides you with an introduction to understanding and undertaking a meta-analysis, which you may like to consider for your own systematic review if appropriate to your review.

1

What is a systematic review?

Overview

- Why do we need systematic reviews in nursing?
- What is a systematic review?
- What is the purpose of systematic reviews within nursing practice?
- How difficult is it to undertake a systematic review?
- What is the role of systematic reviews within evidence-based nursing practice?
- What is the difference between a literature (narrative) review and a systematic review?
- What is the difference between a systematic review and a meta-analysis?
- What are the different types of reviews that can be found in the literature?
- Where can I find systematic reviews?
- What are the drawbacks and limitations of systematic reviews?

Why do we need systematic reviews in nursing?

The original founder of the evidence-based movement emerged from the early works of Archie Cochrane, a Scottish physician and epidemiologist, in the 1960s. A picture of Professor Archibald Leman Cochrane as a composite of hundreds of photos of Cochrane contributors can be found at Cochrane Community (2024). More information about Archie Cochrane can be found on Wikpedia (2023).

Cochrane's concerns were that healthcare providers failed to evaluate the quality and effectiveness of their own practice. Cochrane argued that there was a need for widespread access to scientific literature in order to improve clinical care. Evidence-based medicine, in this context, places less value on authoritative opinion and raises the value of data-based studies and research critiques. The notion of valuing evidence over authoritative opinion initially created controversy and confusion within the profession because of the proposed change. Essentially Cochrane and his colleagues who established the principles of evidence-based medicine firmly believed that sound medicine should focus on:

- demonstrating the potential risks and benefits of medical interventions and practices
- using comprehensive searches to find relevant research

- utilizing randomized controlled trials (RCTs), which are defined as 'the gold standard for effectiveness' (Hariton and Locascio 2018)
- systematic reviews, which are the process of systematically locating, appraising and synthesizing evidence from scientific studies in order to obtain a reliable overview of the best evidence.

It is easy to understand from the above why Cochrane's case for evidence-based medicine was regarded by some colleagues with much cynicism, and even viewed as extremism. This is because at the time his ideas were perceived by peers to be proposing radical changes to existing medical education and medical practice. At this point in time, the quality of research was not necessarily considered and prioritized by practising doctors. The notion of engaging with and applying high-quality evidence like RCTs and systematic reviews was almost alien at the time.

Astonishingly, it took over 30 years for Cochrane's work to be recognized and rewarded in 1992. This was through the establishment of the Cochrane Collaboration, named after Archie Cochrane. The founders, Dr Iain Chalmers, Dr Murray Enkin and Dr Marc Keirse, undertook a comprehensive and painstaking systematic review of all RCTs in the perinatal field. ('Perinatal' refers to the period of time surrounding birth.) The findings, published in 1989, indisputably informed medical practice through the publication of the 'Guide to Effective Care in Pregnancy and Childbirth', detailed below. More significantly, they applauded Cochrane's ideals, recognizing the importance of his work by establishing the Cochrane Collaboration, known today simply as Cochrane (Box 1.1).

Box 1.1   The distinctive symbol of Cochrane

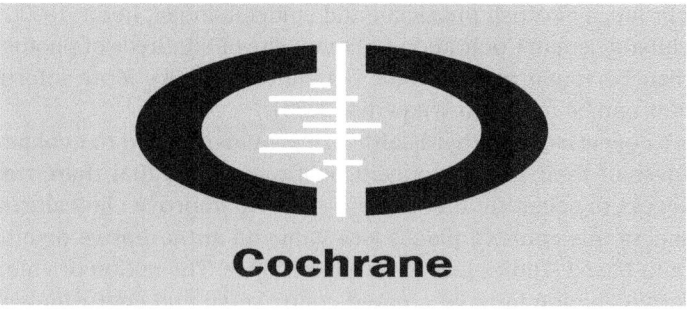

Cochrane, housed at McMaster University, Canada, is a worldwide enterprise with several international centres across various branches. It has been designed specifically around three common goals:

1. Producing trusted evidence
2. Advocating for evidence
3. Informing health and care decisions.

(Cochrane 2023)

In brief, Cochrane comprises a series of review and method groups, centres and consumer networks, designed with the sole purpose of searching for, collecting, reviewing and disseminating the findings from RCTs and systematic reviews. Since the publication of the first Cochrane Database of Systematic Reviews (CDSR) in 1995, the Cochrane Collaboration has continued to grow exponentially year on year, from approximately 65 reviews in 1996 to over 7,500 in 2023 (Cochrane Database of Systematic Reviews 2023).

In 1996 many healthcare professionals were unaware of the profound influence that Cochrane's work would play in changing the way medical education and practice (indeed all health and social care) is provided. Although unnoticed and unrecognized at the time, Cochrane was, in essence, laying down the foundations of the evidence-based movement of today. Rycroft-Malone et al. (2004) believe that, since its conception, the term 'evidence-based' has swept across the world like a new pandemic, evolving as the dominant theme of practice, policy, management, education and research within health and social care services. Cochrane's landmark work – identifying the principles and processes associated with evidence-based medicine – and the subsequent endorsement of the term by McMaster University have led to it becoming the 'mantra' of the movement.

Strikingly, a series of incremental steps, founded on Cochrane's 1979 seminal work, highlight how the term 'evidence-based' has evolved to become universally professionally desirable and acceptable. These include, for example, evidence-based medicine (Sackett et al. 1996), evidence-based nursing (DiCenso et al. 1998) and evidence-based practice (Muir Gray 1997).

Parallel to the expanding uni-professional evidence-based terms, the relative merits and demerits of engaging with the 'evidence' have resulted in a broadening of the term. The term now incorporates evidence-based practice (DiCenso et al. 1998), evidence-based practice and rehabilitation (Tse et al. 2004) and evidence-based occupational therapy (Law and Baum 1998). Youngblut and Brooten (2001) suggest that the term 'evidence-based' aims to ensure that Cochrane's principles extend beyond health and social care professionals to the wider managerial, administrative and educational settings. The potential advantages and disadvantages of engaging with an evidence base have become so important that the whole of the health and social care spectrum has been included under the generic banner we term 'evidence-based health and social care'. Interestingly, these terms, collectively, have become known as the evidence-based movement (Greenhalgh et al. 2014).

The evidence-based movement can be described as the coming together of several fundamental elements designed to maximize both the performance and outcomes of individual(s), systems and processes. According to Greenhalgh et al. (2018) and Kumah et al. 2022) these include, but are not restricted to:

- accessing, reviewing and synthesizing best available published evidence via systematic reviews and in some instances with meta-analyses and synthesis
- informing clinical judgement and decision-making, with the best evidence
- ensuring patient needs and desires are integrated within the decision-making processes
- working within the scope and practices surrounding professional accountability (i.e. safety, quality, governance and outcomes).

Historically not all nursing practices, interventions and treatments were underpinned by quality evidence; in some instances they were based upon rituals and traditions. You may have heard the phrase 'This is the way we have always done things around here', suggesting possible resistance to changing the way things were done in the past. Both the resistance and challenges to change have led to a drive for nursing care to become evidence based. The importance of systematic reviews, we would suggest, is enshrined within the evidence-based movement. This is due, primarily but not exclusively, to the reasons illustrated in Figure 1.1. The drivers in Figure 1.1 can be categorized into several broad themes: political, professional, societal, economical and personal.

Systematic reviews undoubtably contribute to the evidence base for nurses to use in supporting their decisions and actions in nursing practice. The interchangeable nature of the drivers for evidence demonstrates its importance for ensuring safety, quality and care. The drivers reveal the complexities and interconnectedness of getting evidence into practice, because suboptimal and substandard care and services are no longer acceptable. Professional regulators are reaffirming the need for the

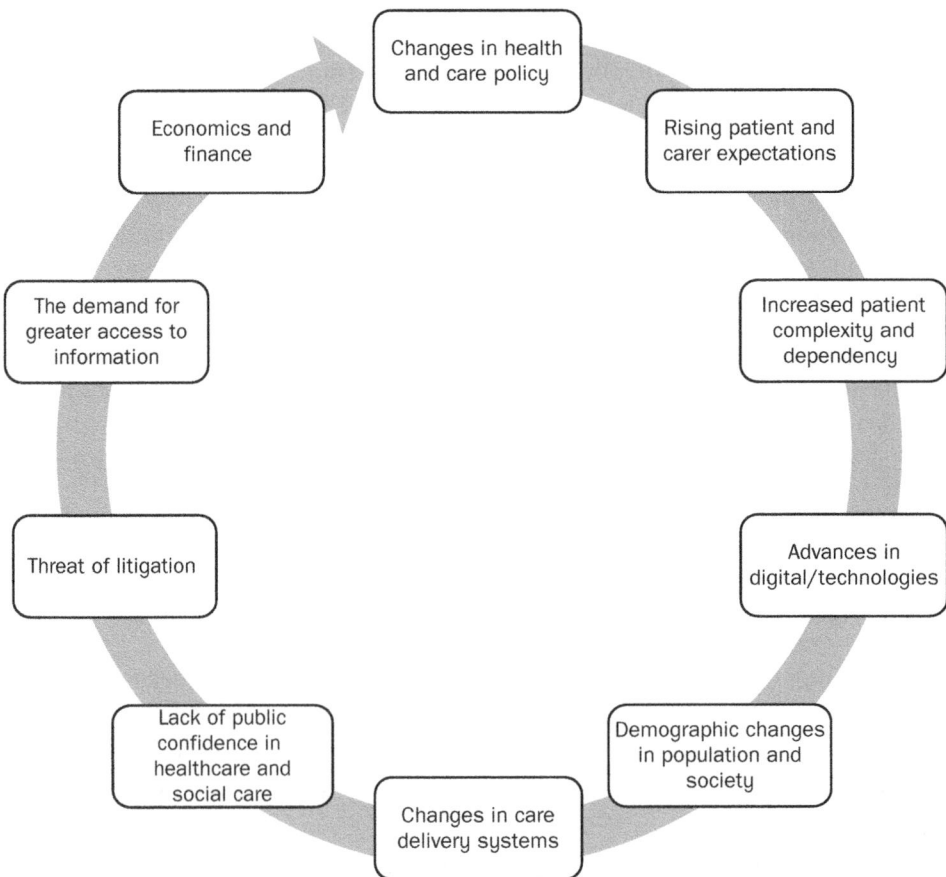

Figure 1.1 Drivers for systematic reviews within the evidence-based movement.

application of the best available evidence. The challenge facing nurses is in defining what comprises a systematic review, how you engage with the various processes and how you can share and disseminate the findings.

> ### Practical Tip
>
> Since the creation of the Cochrane organization, several other establishments have emerged focusing on high-quality evidence through systematic reviews. Examples of these are provided in Box 1.2 on p. 20 in the section 'Where can I find systematic reviews?'

What is a systematic review?

A systematic review is a synthesis (mixture, amalgam, fusion) of the research literature that is focused on answering a single question. We use the term 'synthesis' as opposed to 'summary' (which we applied in the previous edition) to illustrate the following differences. Synthesis is the overall coming together of the review's processes, drawing out the critical findings from the various research articles to form a whole picture to answer the question. Summary, on the other hand, is essentially a synopsis (precis, resume, outline) of the systematic review's findings and outcomes that can be shared and disseminated.

A systematic review is conducted in a manner that tries to identify, select, appraise and synthesize all high-quality research evidence relevant to that question. High-quality research includes those studies with an explicit and rigorous design that allows the findings to be interrogated against clear contexts and research intentions. When conducting systematic reviews, we need to accept that there is a hierarchy of evidence and that what can confidently be stated *empirically* (by observation and experience) about the world is derived from studies where the design is both explicit and rigorous. Distinctions therefore need to be made about the type of research approach adopted – that is, quantitative (numbers), qualitative (experience) or mixed methods. The latter is a combination of both qualitative and quantitative approaches. Irrespective of the type of research approach used, this should be rigorously reviewed and scrutinized. Synthesis is about 'translating': the process of moving the findings into words, texts and languages so that they can be used in different countries, cultures, contexts and places. Translation is essential for: a) sharing and disseminating the findings to enable b) the application of evidence to inform decision-making – a highly important step that is often ignored. An overview of a systematic review is provided in Figure 1.2 on p. 6.

Having an understanding of systematic reviews and how to implement them in practice is mandatory for all nurses and other healthcare professionals as part of standards for professional practice (HCPC n.d.; NMC n.d.)

You will find that there are numerous definitions of systematic reviews available. These definitions range from a brief sentence to several paragraphs. You may also note that these definitions have evolved over time to:

- streamline both the systems and processes
- clarify the individual steps involved

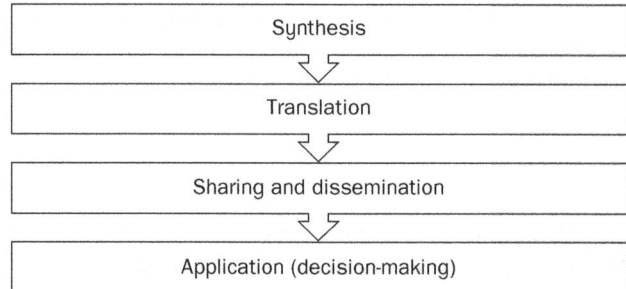

Figure 1.2 Overview of a systematic review.

- highlight databases to enable the management of data (primary papers that meet your systematic review criteria)
- provide various sources and resources to aid you in doing your systematic review.

Table 1.1 also illustrates how views on systematic reviews have evolved over time, highlighting the various steps and associated systems and processes required to conduct a high-quality review. As illustrated in Figure 1.3, we would suggest that, over

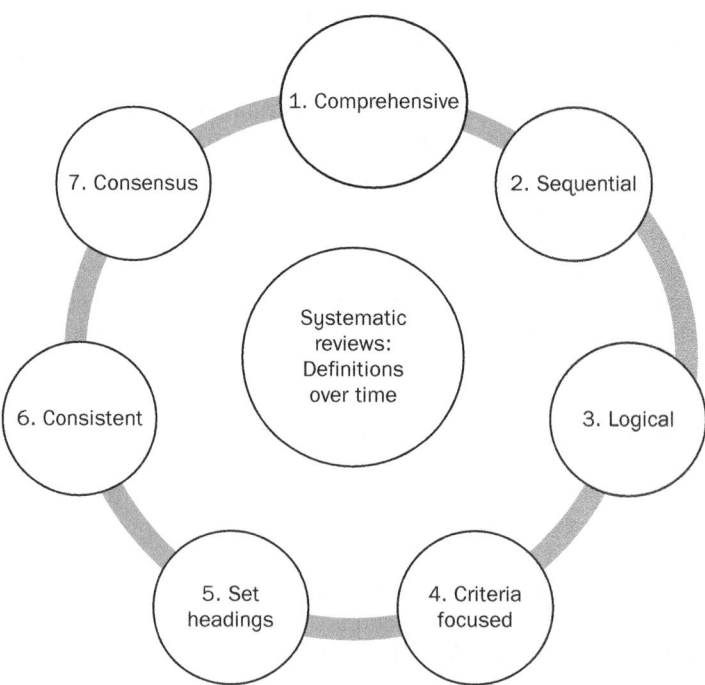

Figure 1.3 Evolution of systematic review definitions over time.

Table 1.1 Definitions of the concept 'systematic review' from 2009 to 2022, in chronological order

Year	Source	Definition	Key themes	Authors' observations
2009	CRD (Centre for Reviews and Dissemination) (2009: v)	'Health care decisions for individual patients and for public policy should be informed by the best available research evidence. Practitioners and decision-makers are encouraged to make use of the latest research and information about best practice, and to ensure that decisions are demonstrably rooted in this knowledge.'	• Healthcare decision-making for patients • Best available evidence • Best practice • Knowledge application	The emphasis is on professional orientation. Patients are mentioned but they seem to be disconnected from the definition. They are not the main focus.
2011	Clarke (2011: 64)	'A systematic review uses all the existing research and is sometime called "secondary research" (research on research). They are often required by research funders to establish the state of existing knowledge and are frequently used in guideline development.'	• All existing research • State of knowledge • Guideline development	This reaffirms the importance of systematic reviews in looking at all existing research knowledge and that they should inform guideline and policy development.
2013	Gopalakrishnan and Ganeshkumar (2013: 9)	'Systematic reviews aim to identify, evaluate and summarise the findings of all relevant individual studies, thereby making the available evidence more accessible to decision makers.'	• Purpose and processes • Synthesis • Accessibility • Decision-making	There is a strong focus on the purposes and processes of doing a systematic review and the importance of synthesizing and making evidence accessible for decision-makers. There is no reference to patients or joint decision-making.

(Continued)

Table 1.1 *(Continued)*

Year	Source	Definition	Key themes	Authors' observations
2022	NIHR (National Institute for Health and Care Research) (2022)	'A review of a clearly formulated question that uses systematic and explicit methods to identify, select, and critically appraise relevant research, and to collect and analyse data from the studies that are included in the review. Statistical methods (meta-analysis) may or may not be used to analyse and summarise the results of the included studies	• Identification of a problem and development of a question • System and processes of doing the systematic review • Highlights the importance of statistical data and results	This reaffirms the importance of problem identification and how this should inform the development of the question, engagement with the systems and processes and appropriate data and statistical analysis.
2022	The Cochrane Handbook, Chapter 1 (Higgins et al. 2022: n.p.)	'Systematic reviews seek to collate evidence that fits pre-specified eligibility criteria in order to answer a specific research question. They aim to minimize bias by using explicit, systematic methods documented in advance with a protocol.'	• Collection of evidence set against a predetermined research question and criteria • Systems and processes of undertaking a comprehensive review	This highlights the importance of having sound, robust criteria to help inform the framing of the systematic review question. The terms 'systems' and 'processes' reaffirm the importance of having well-defined eligibility criteria to follow, in order to strengthen your systematic review and to minimize bias.

Table 1.1 (*Continued*)

Year	Source	Definition	Key themes	Authors' observations
2022	Joanna Briggs Institute (Santos et al. 2018: n.p.)	'Systematic reviews aim to provide a comprehensive, unbiased synthesis of many relevant studies in a single document using rigorous and transparent methods. A systematic review aims to synthesize and summarize existing knowledge. It attempts to uncover "all" of the evidence relevant to a question.'	• Systems, processes and methods to undertake a comprehensive review • Synthesis • Knowledge • Evidence aligned to a specific review question	This reaffirms the importance of having sound systems and processes/ methods in order to undertake a quality systematic review. Synthesis of existing knowledge is imperative to identify any gaps in the evidence. A quality systematic review should aim to identify all evidence relevant to your review question.
2022	CRD (2022)	'Definitions vary but high quality reviews usually aim to answer a research question by: • identifying all relevant published and unpublished evidence on the subject of the review • selecting studies for inclusion • assessing the quality of every included study • synthesising the findings from all of the studies in an unbiased way • presenting a balanced summary of the findings.'	Answering a specific research question through the application of a set series of systems and processes	A comprehensive set of systems and processes is necessary to guide the systematic review. Your ability to answer a specific research question would be compromised if you don't have a robust set of criteria and guidelines to follow. A structured review minimizes bias or avoids the introduction of bias.

time, the definitions have become more comprehensive, sequential, logical and criteria focused, with set headings, offering both consistency and consensus in the definition of what a systematic review is and how to carry out a systematic review.

In our opinion, based on the critique provided in Table 1.1, a high-quality systematic review can be regarded as a:

> working framework comprising of a series of logical, criteria-focused, sequential steps designed to address a specific review question. The question is aimed at addressing a clinical, educational, managerial, business or engineering topic or area/s within a field and specialty-specific discipline. Emphasis needs to be placed on identifying all published and unpublished literature relevant to the review question. This is followed by selecting studies for inclusion, assessing the quality of every chosen study, extracting and synthesizing data from each included study (for some quantitative systematic reviews, statistical methods such as meta-analysis may be undertaken). Finally, an unbiased summary of the findings is presented. The evidence should be used to inform decision-making by individual nurses and midwives, in partnership with patients, regarding the utilization and application of this evidence in meeting their preferences to the benefit of the patient, family and healthcare professional and in terms of safety and quality. The utilization of the evidence is dependent on having a sound sharing and dissemination strategy (in other words, if you do not communicate your findings, people will not become aware of them).

In our opinion several limitations in the various definitions detailed in Table 1.1 require further clarification in demonstrating how they have contributed to informing nurses and midwives as well as the profession's utilization and application of evidence in practice. There seems to be an implicit acceptance within the definitions that evidence is used to inform shared decision-making with patients, service users or the public, together with the evidence of their preference or choices. However, this is not explicitly articulated. We would suggest that the outcomes of systematic reviews should be more specific in detailing how they may inform patient choice and decision-making, alongside improving safety and quality of care and services. The knowledge generated requires translating into simple language for patients to understand. This can only be achieved by having a robust sharing and dissemination strategy.

Practical Tip

A systematic review is a framework within which high-quality evidence is generated through a comprehensive, logical, sequential series of systematic processes. A systematic review *is not evidence-based nursing on its own*. A systematic review is only a component of evidence-based nursing in that it facilitates the generation of best available knowledge as evidence.

What is the purpose of systematic reviews within nursing practice?

The Centre for Reviews and Dissemination (CRD) at the University of York (2009: v) suggests that the purpose of systematic reviews is as follows:

> Health care decisions for individual patients and for public policy should be informed by the best available research evidence. Practitioners and decision-makers are encouraged to make use of the latest research and information about best practice, and to ensure that decisions are demonstrably rooted in this knowledge.

However, operationalizing the above definition can sometimes be difficult for nurses, midwives and researchers because of the seemingly infinite volume of information that is continually being published in a multitude of journals worldwide. Individual research studies may also be biased or methodologically unsound and can reach conflicting conclusions. Examples of conflicting research results are frequently found in the media, which may announce, for instance, that based on the research results of the latest study the contraceptive pill is 'safe', and then a week later proclaim the exact opposite based on the results of another research study. In such situations it is not always clear which results are the most reliable, or which should be used as the basis of individual, policy and practice decisions (Purssell and McCrae 2020).

A systematic review should be based on a peer-review protocol (or plan) so that it can be easily replicated if necessary. The review itself will include a 'background' or 'introduction', in which the authors explain the scientific context for their study. It also includes the rationale for the systematic review, indicating why it is necessary. The specific objectives and a summary of how the reviewer defined the criteria by which to choose the research papers are stated. Once a thorough assessment of the quality of each included research paper has been carried out, all the individual studies are synthesized in an unbiased way. The findings are then interpreted and presented in an objective and independent summary.

Systematic reviews are used by a wide diversity of professional and non-professional groups, including not only doctors, nurses and other healthcare professionals but also service users, policymakers, researchers, lecturers and students who want to keep abreast of the evidence in their field. It is important that nurses and midwives have the research knowledge, skills and competence to both understand and undertake systematic reviews. This is because they may want to know the answer to a clinical or research question or they may be conducting a systematic review as part of a dissertation required to complete a degree or as continuing professional development. Conducting a systematic review can initially appear to be an epic task, but once the steps of the process are learnt, and provided enough time is set aside, the task is relatively straightforward.

We would suggest that, based on the above, the primary purposes of undertaking a systematic review can be broken down into several categories, namely evidence, policy, profession and outcomes (EPPO):

Evidence:
1   To increase the knowledge and evidence base for nurses and other health and social care professions

Policy:

2   To inform policy development and decision-making by individuals, patients, organizations and the profession(s)

Profession:

3   To enhance the understanding of the profession

4   To improve shared decision-making between nurses, patients and professionals

Outcomes:

5   To ensure the best treatments and interventions are used, that they provide efficient and effective outcomes and are value for money

6   To improve safety, quality, standards and care

7   To enhance the quality of the clinical teaching and learning environment (CTLE) for students and staff.

How difficult is it to undertake a systematic review?

Having taught large numbers of students on dissertation modules about how to conduct a systematic review, we are confident that both undergraduate and postgraduate students can competently undertake and complete this type of review to a satisfactory level. If this is the first time you are undertaking a systematic review, remember the following:

1   Allow sufficient time to plan and work on all the stages of the systematic review.

2   Ensure that you carry out the review methodically, as detailed, following each step.

3   Complete each step, taking enough time to do them comprehensively. This will help increase both your confidence and your standard of work.

Practical Tip

A systematic review can only be undertaken using primary research papers. It is not possible to conduct a systematic review using other types of studies such as narrative reviews or opinion papers.

The three main types of systematic reviews are *quantitative, qualitative* and *mixed-method* reviews. Quantitative systematic reviews generally include only quantitative primary research studies, whereas qualitative systematic reviews include only qualitative primary research studies. Mixed-method reviews are based on both qualitative and quantitative studies; they are becoming more popular, although they may be a bit more difficult to conduct. Further information on conducting a mixed-methods systematic review is available at the following:

Stern, C., Lizarondo, L., Carrier, J., et al. (2020) Methodological guidance for the conduct of mixed methods systematic reviews. *JBI Evidence Synthesis* 10: 2108–2118.

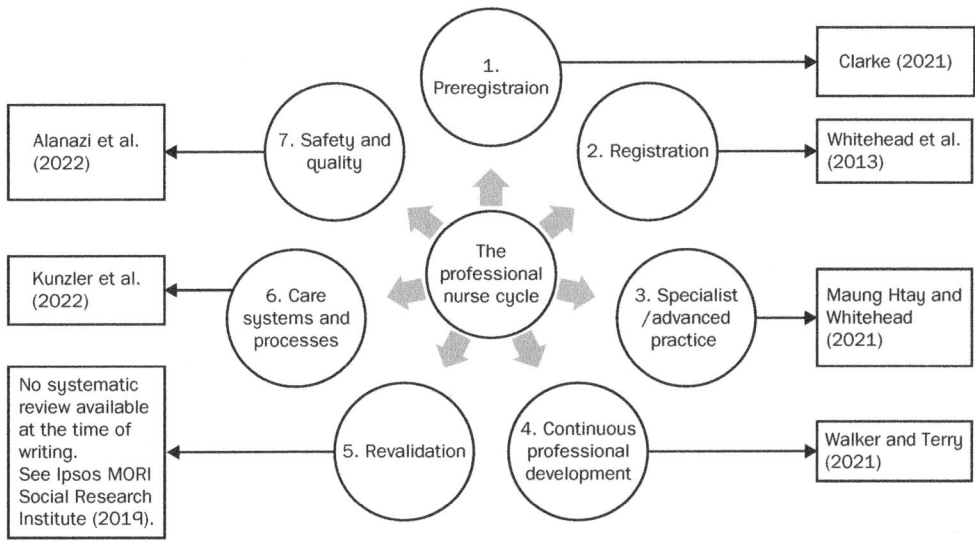

Figure 1.4 The evolution of systematic reviews in nursing around the professional nurse cycle.

For the sake of simplicity, this book will consider only the quantitative and qualitative types of systematic reviews.

There are several sources available for finding systematic reviews, as detailed in Box 1.2, whether quantitative, qualitative or mixed methods. It is also important to highlight that apart from the Campbell Collaboration and the Cochrane Library, many systematic reviews are published in key professional nursing and health and care journals.

Since the publication of the first (2012) and second (2016) editions of our book, over what is a relatively short period of time, the number of systematic reviews both undertaken and published in nursing has increased exponentially. Figure 1.4 illustrates the evolution of systematic reviews around what we have termed the professional nurse cycle (PNC).

According to Figure 1.4, by targeting the key attributes of becoming, maintaining and revalidating your registration to practise as a nurse, it is possible to highlight the emergence of the professional nurse cycle. For example, in the UK, when you commence an undergraduate preregistration nurse education programme, this leads to registration as a professional nurse, which you must maintain through continuous professional development and revalidation every three years. More detailed information is offered in Table 1.2 on p. 14.

Table 1.2 illustrates the seven components of the PNC and offers an example of a systematic review for each component, apart from number 5, for which a systematic review was unavailable at the time of writing. We would suggest that when you begin to think about your systematic review in nursing, you may wish to reflect upon areas aligned to the PNC – that is, the systems and processes of clinical practice – nursing, education (other fields) – and safety, quality of care and services and how these may

Table 1.2 Unpicking the professional nurse cycle

PNC sequence and label	Rationale	Examples of systematic review to corroborate the PNC
1: Preregistration	Undergraduate preregistration nurse education is about acquiring the knowledge, skills, confidence and competence to perform the role responsibly, effectively and safely.	Clarke (2021)
2: Registration	To become a registered nurse, you are required to have successfully completed the standards and competences set out by a validated programme of study by a recognized nursing regulator or professional body.	Whitehead et al. (2013)
3: Specialist/ advanced practice	To become a specialist or advanced nurse you are required to have successfully completed a recognized programme of study approved by a nursing regulator or professional body.	Maung Htay and Whitehead (2021)
4: Continuous professional development	Continuous professional development is essential to advance and retain your professional knowledge, competency and confidence and in supporting you to deliver safe, quality care.	Walker and Terry (2021)
5: Revalidation	To remain on a professional nursing register, you are required to demonstrate that you have updated and maintained your knowledge, skills and competency through completing a revalidation programme. These tend to be every three years. Failure to complete the revalidation process could result in your removal from the register to practice.	Ipsos MORI Social Research Institute (2019)
6: Care systems and processes	Care systems and processes are essentially the mechanisms that enable structures, technologies and people to work together efficiently and effectively. This is achieved by bringing together the key stakeholders and partners associated with the delivery of health and care organizations, local authorities and others. These take collective responsibility for planning services and improving health and well-being by reducing inequalities across local geographical areas.	Kunzler et al. (2022)
7: Safety and quality	The delivery of safe, quality care and services is the primary aim and responsibility of all health and care systems and processes.	Alanazi et al. (2022)

impact on patient outcomes. For example, you could focus on the enabling and inhibiting factors aligned to the delivery of person-centred care and/or the type of care, place and location where care takes place – primary care, secondary care, acute care, home care, and so forth. It is also worth noting that the PNC may be influenced by the workplace and organizational culture, as well as by the environment in which you work. For example, having insufficient time, support and resources to undertake continuous professional development, revalidation activities and/or a systematic review will have an impact. Focusing on the PNC may help to stimulate your ideas for generating a research question, discussed in Chapter 2.

Practical Tip

Systematic reviews are a sound way of keeping up to date with the latest evidence surrounding a specific area and aspect of nursing. Systematic reviews are regularly updated and are current sources of evidence.

What is the role of systematic reviews within evidence-based nursing practice?

As previously mentioned in the section 'Why do we need systematic reviews in nursing?', the popularity of evidence-based practice has increased significantly since the mid-1990s, when Sackett et al. (1996) coined the term. DiCenso et al. (1998: 38) comment that in order to practice evidence-based nursing,

> A nurse has to decide whether the evidence is relevant for the particular patient. The incorporation of clinical expertise should be balanced with the risks and benefits of alternative treatments for each patient and should take into account the patient's unique clinical circumstances including comorbid conditions and preferences.

It is important to think about what is meant by the *best* research evidence. Within evidence-based practice there is a hierarchy of research evidence relating to studies with different types of research designs. This hierarchy has systematic reviews at the top and qualitative studies and opinion papers towards the bottom (Table 1.3). The hierarchy of evidence is a medically based model that is considered by some professional groups to be biased towards quantitative research and intervention studies. Although qualitative studies are found at the bottom, it is important to consider that they answer very different types of questions relating to patient experiences. A few authors and researchers have objected to the classification in Table 1.3, stating that this model does not accurately represent the high-quality qualitative research studies that inform policy and practice and that perhaps better represent patient experiences and preferences.

The traditional scientific approach to finding the best research evidence is to carry out or read a literature review (conducted by an expert or well-known figure in the field). However, these traditional (or narrative) reviews, even those written by

Table 1.3 Levels of evidence for different types of research questions

Level 1a	A well-conducted systematic review of RCTs
Level 1b	One good-quality RCT
Level 1c	All or none
Level 2a	Systematic review of cohort studies
Level 2b	One cohort study
Level 2c	Outcomes research, i.e. the effect of an intervention or treatment
Level 3a	Systematic review of case-control studies
Level 3b	Case series
Level 4	One case study
Level 5	Systematic review of descriptive, qualitative studies
Level 6	Single descriptive or qualitative study
Level 7	Expert opinion, reports of expert committees, quality improvement reports, evidence-based practice projects

Note: The research questions can include nursing interventions, therapy, prevention, aetiology (causes) or harm.

experts, can be made to tell any story one wants them to, and failure by literature reviewers to apply scientific principles to the process of reviewing, just as one would to primary research, can lead to biased conclusions, harm to patients and wasted resources (Petticrew and Roberts 2006: 5).

Craig and Dowding (2019) suggest that a systematic review should include a detailed search strategy, a review and a synthesis of the included articles, which also aligns with the principles of evidence-based practice.

Systematic reviews provide practitioners with a way of gaining access to predigested evidence. According to Petticrew and Roberts (2006: 9), systematic reviews 'adhere closely to a set of scientific methods that explicitly aim to limit systematic error (bias), mainly attempting to identify, appraise and synthesize all relevant studies (of whatever design) in order *to answer a particular question (or set of questions)*' (our emphasis). Systematic reviews substantially reduce the time and expertise it would take to locate, appraise and synthesize individual studies.

What is the difference between a literature (narrative) review and a systematic review?

Traditional literature (narrative) reviews can, as already mentioned, tell any story that the reviewer wants them to (Glasziou et al. 2001). For example, if the reviewer is a strong believer in the effectiveness of aspirin for treating headaches but does not believe that any other medication is effective, this reviewer could (hypothetically) select all the papers showing the effectiveness of aspirin and leave out all the ones showing the effectiveness of, say, ibuprofen.

While both traditional (narrative) and systematic reviews provide summaries of the available literature on a topic, they fulfill very different needs. Although narrative reviews (also called critical reviews) provide valuable summaries by experts on a wide topic area, they usually present an *overview*. These types of reviews do not usually follow a scientific review methodology and the papers included can be haphazard and biased. Nevertheless, they can be an important source of ideas, arguments, context and information. Narrative reviews are valuable because they are written by experts in the field and provide a general summary of the topic area, but they may not always include all the literature on the topic and sometimes they may be biased in terms of which articles are selected and discussed (Petticrew and Roberts 2006).

Narrative reviewers can be influenced by their preferred theories, needs and beliefs. It is important to remember that narrative reviews are usually driven by a general interest in a topic and *not* directed by a stated question. Narrative reviews do not state the criteria that determine the search undertaken and can be disorganized. A notorious example is the review conducted by the eminent doctor Linus Pauling (1974), who was a Nobel Prize laureate. In 1974, having conducted a non-systematic traditional review, he concluded that people should be getting 100 times the amount of vitamin C that the food and nutrition board recommended at the time; he suggested that such doses could *prevent* a cold. Some 30 years later Douglas et al. (2004) conducted a thorough Cochrane systematic review of papers from the same period as Pauling's review; they concluded that high doses of vitamin C *did not prevent* colds (although it could reduce the duration by one or two days). Douglas et al. (2004) found that Pauling had failed to include 15 relevant studies in his review. It is therefore important to remember that 'a haphazard review, even one carried out by an expert, can be misleading' (Petticrew and Roberts 2006: 6).

A systematic review, in contrast, uses *a comprehensive rigorous research methodology* to try to limit bias in all aspects of the review. In this sense it is close to a primary research study, where the participants are not people but rather the papers included in the review. Khan and Zamora (2022) support evidence-based practice through the use of case studies and explore how to appraise, conduct and publish a systematic review. Table 1.4 summarizes the differences and similarities between the two types of reviews.

What is the difference between a systematic review and a meta-analysis?

As described above, a systematic review is a thorough, comprehensive and explicit way of evaluating the nursing literature. It is a summary of the research literature that is focused on a single question. It is conducted in a manner that tries to identify, select, appraise and synthesize all high-quality research evidence relevant to that question. A systematic review may or may not include a meta-analysis.

A meta-analysis is a statistical approach to combine the data derived from a systematic review. Therefore, every meta-analysis should be based on an underlying systematic review, but not every systematic review leads to a meta-analysis. For more information see Chapter 13.

Table 1.4 Similarities and differences between a narrative review and a systematic review

	Systematic reviews	*Narrative reviews*
Question	Focused on a single question	Not necessarily focused on a single question but may describe an overview of a topic
Protocol	A peer-review protocol (or plan) is included	No protocol
Background/literature review	Both provide summaries of the available literature on a topic	
Objectives	Clear objectives stated	Objectives may or may not be identified
Inclusion/exclusion criteria	Criteria stated before the review is conducted	Criteria not usually specified
Search strategy	Comprehensive search conducted in a systematic way	Search strategy not explicitly stated
Process of selecting papers	Selection process usually clear and explicit	Selection process not described
Process of evaluating papers	Comprehensive evaluation of study quality	Evaluation of study quality may or may not be included
Process of extracting relevant information	Process is usually clear and specific	Process of extracting relevant information is not explicit and clear
Results/data synthesis	Clear summaries of studies based on high-quality evidence	Summary based on studies where the quality of included papers may not be specified, and can be influenced by reviewers' pet theories, needs and beliefs
Discussion	Written by an expert or group of experts with a detailed and well-grounded knowledge of the issues	
Sharing and dissemination	Designing a detailed strategic plan outlining how and where you intend to share and disseminate your findings and recommendations is essential	

What are the different types of reviews that can be found in the literature?

Table 1.5 details the different types of reviews that can be found in the literature.

Table 1.5 Different types of reviews found in the literature

Label	Description
Comprehensive systematic review	The highest level of evidence, associated with following a highly a comprehensive series of steps and processes to elicit the best evidence
Rapid review	A brief version of a systematic review to search and critically appraise existing research
Scoping review	A brief review, the aim of which is to identify the potential size and scope of the available research literature
Critical review	A term usually used interchangeably with the term 'narrative review'
Mixed-studies review or mixed-methods review	Combines both quantitative and qualitative reviewing, to produce the systematic review
Qualitative systematic review/qualitative evidence synthesis	Synthesizes the findings from qualitative studies; looks for trends across individual qualitative studies
Overview	Summary of the (medical) literature that attempts to survey the literature and describe its characteristics
Umbrella review	Synthesis and summary of evidence from a group of reviews
Aggregative review	Reviews are synthesized by adding up (aggregating/counting) data to answer review questions
Configurative review	Associated with organizing and arranging data. These are usually but not always associated with qualitative data; in some instances, quantitative data can be organized and configured too
Integrative review	Associated with the types of studies included in the review
Quick and dirty review	A simple approach that enables you to identify and document relevant information in an organized and intentional format
Mixed-methods review	A combination of both qualitative and quantitative primary research studies

Where can I find systematic reviews?

Systematic reviews can be found in several different nursing journals and on specialist websites. Box 1.2 provides some useful websites to start searching for systematic reviews.

Box 1.2 Websites for finding systematic reviews

Campbell Collaboration	https://www.campbellcollaboration.org/
Cochrane Library	www.thecochranelibrary.com
Centre for Reviews and Dissemination (CRD), University of York	www.york.ac.uk/crd/
Evidence-Based Nursing (EBN) (journal)	http://ebn.bmj.com/
Evidence for Policy and Practice Information and Co-ordinating Centre (EPPI Centre)	http://eppi.ioe.ac.uk/cms/Default. aspx?tabid=63
Joanna Briggs Institute	https://jbi.global/
National Health Service (NHS), Health Education England, Knowledge and Library Services: Resources for Advanced Searching	https://library.nhs.uk/knowledgehub/ resources-for-advanced-searching/
Sheffield Centre for Health and Related Research (SCHARR), University of Sheffield	https://www.sheffield.ac.uk/scharr
Systematic Reviews (journal)	https://systematicreviewsjournal. biomedcentral.com/
TRIP database	www.tripdatabase.com
Cochrane Qualitative & Implementation Methods Group	https://methods.cochrane.org/qi/
CINAHL database and CINAHL complete	https://www.ebscohost.com/academic/ cinahl-plus-with-full-text
Worldviews on Evidence-based Nursing (journal)	http://onlinelibrary.wiley.com/ journal/10.1111/(ISSN)1741-6787

In the UK, the UK Cochrane Centre supports the preparation of systematic reviews of the effects of healthcare interventions produced by numerous Cochrane Review Groups funded by the National Institute for Health and Care Research (NIHR). As it suggests on the website, the systematic reviews are regularly updated to ensure that treatment decisions are based on the best up-to-date and reliable evidence (http://community.cochrane.org/cochrane-reviews). Other databases where systematic reviews as well as ongoing reviews can be registered are found at the following:

- Prospero is an open access international prospective register of systematic reviews in health and social care, available at https://www.crd.york.ac.uk/PROSPERO/.

- The Health Technology Assessment programme collates information on completed and ongoing health technology assessments from numerous international agencies. The reviews independently assess the existing evidence based on the benefits, harm and costs of particular healthcare treatments and tests for those who plan, provide or receive care in the National Health Service (NHS). Further information is available at https://www.nihr.ac.uk/explore-nihr/funding-programmes/health-technology-assessment.htm.

- The CRD previously maintained access to the Database of Abstracts of Reviews of Effects (DARE) and the NHS Economic Evaluation Database (NHS EED). These databases contain quality assessed systematic reviews and economic evaluations of health and social care interventions that have been published. These databases are currently available via the International HTA Database at https://database.inahta.org/.

What are the drawbacks and limitations of systematic reviews?

Although systematic reviews can be found at the top of the hierarchy of evidence, this does not mean that we should always believe the results presented within them. Like any other piece of research, a systematic review can be conducted badly, so it is important to have the skills to be able to appraise them (see Chapters 6–12). Systematic reviews may also be biased in the way the papers are selected, for instance if they have not included all the primary research papers available. Sometimes systematic reviews include only English-language papers and ignore all non-English-language papers, which may have found different results.

Other types of biases can occur in the way that reviewers search for their research papers. If the reviewers did not conduct a comprehensive search drawing on the most relevant databases, searching for grey literature and hand searching, it is possible that a number of key papers may have been left out. Furthermore, systematic reviews may fail to properly combine the results of different studies and so end up presenting inaccurate results.

It is crucial to appraise a systematic review properly before using the results. To do this you need to ask a series of questions to evaluate if the review in question conducted all the steps in the process correctly and with minimal bias.

🗝 Key points

- Having a comprehensive understanding of why and how the evidence-based movement originated and its influence on systematic reviews is essential.

- Systematic reviews are regarded as a key element of evidence-based nursing that may impact change within clinical practice, research, policy and economics.

- A systematic review is a research article that identifies a specific review question, identifies all relevant studies, appraises their quality and summarizes their results using a scientific methodology.

- It is possible to conduct systematic reviews of many different types of primary research studies.
- Sources for finding systematic reviews include the Cochrane Library, the Campbell Collaboration, the Cochrane Qualitative Research Group and key nursing journals, among others.
- Systematic reviews are based on research evidence and the synthesis of research studies and can also be used to inform important policies that affect both the quality and the safety and value of health and care.
- Because systematic reviews include a comprehensive search strategy, appraisal and synthesis of research evidence, they can be used as shortcuts in the evidence-based process.
- Both traditional (narrative) and systematic reviews provide summaries of the available literature on a topic but they fulfill very different needs.
- Narrative reviews provide valuable summaries by experts on a wide topic area and they usually present an *overview*.
- Narrative reviews do not follow a scientific review methodology and the papers included within them can be haphazard and biased, usually influenced by the opinions of the study authors.
- Exploring the PNC may be an aide-memoir in supporting you to identify an area of practice that requires further research via a systematic review.

Summary

This chapter introduced the evidence-based movement and how this relates to the undertaking of a systematic review. A further discussion of the different types of reviews within nursing research and practice was offered and their role within evidence-based nursing practice was explored. The chapter provided different types of databases to help find any relevant systematic reviews and discussed the PNC to help support you in identifying a potential area for a systematic review. The differences between literature (narrative) reviews and systematic reviews were debated and the medical hierarchy of evidence was briefly discussed. The chapter concluded by discussing the drawbacks and limitations of systematic reviews.

Question and Answer (Q&A)

(Q) Why do nurses working on the frontline need to understand about systematic reviews?

(A) Systematic reviews are an excellent way of finding answers to problems. Systematic reviews are a good way of keeping up to date with the latest evidence. They help facilitate the inclusion of evidence into nursing practice.

References

Alanazi, F.K., Sim, J. and Lapkin, S. (2022) Systematic review: Nurses' safety attitudes and their impact on patient outcomes in acute-care hospitals. *Nursing Open* 9 (1): 30–43.

Clarke, H. (2021) How pre-registration nursing students acquire delegation skills: A systematic literature review. *Nurse Education Today* 106: 1–7.

Clarke, J. (2011) What is a systematic review? *Evidence-Based Nursing* 14 (3): 64.

Cochrane (2023) About us. Available at https://www.cochrane.org/about-us (accessed 22 March 2023).

Cochrane Community (2024) Archie Cochrane: The name behind Cochrane. Available at https://community.cochrane.org/archie-cochrane-name-behind-cochrane (accessed 24 February 2024).

Cochrane Database of Systematic Reviews (2023) All issues. Available at https://www.cochranelibrary.com/cdsr/table-of-contents (accessed 22 March 2023).

Craig, J. and Dowding, D. (2019) *The Evidence-Based Practice Manual for Nurses*, 4th edn. London: Churchill Livingstone.

CRD (Centre for Reviews and Dissemination) (2009) *Systematic Reviews: CRD's Guidance for Undertaking Reviews in Health Care*. Available at http://www.york.ac.uk/crd/guidance/ (accessed 26 April 2023).

CRD (Center for Reviews and Dissemination) (2022) Systematic reviews: A practical guide. University of York. Available at https://subjectguides.york.ac.uk/systematic-review/expectations (accessed 9 November 2022).

DiCenso, A., Cullum, N. and Ciliska, D. (1998) Implementing evidence-based nursing: Some misconceptions. *Evidence-Based Nursing* 1: 38–39.

Douglas, R.M., Hemilä, H., Chalker, E. and Treacy, B. (2004) Vitamin C for preventing and treating the common cold. Cochrane Database of Systematic Reviews CD000980. https://doi.org/10.1002/14651858.CD000980.pub4.

Glasziou, P., Irwig, L., Bain, C. and Colditz, G. (2001) *Systematic Reviews in Health Care: A Practical Guide*. Cambridge: Cambridge University Press.

Gopalakrishnan, S. and Ganeshkumar, P. (2013) Systematic reviews and meta-analysis: Understanding the best evidence in primary healthcare. *Journal of Family Medicine and Primary Care* 2 (1): 9–14.

Greenhalgh, T., Howick, J. and Maskrey, N. (2014) Evidence based medicine: A movement in crisis? *British Medical Journal* 13 (348): 3725.

Greenhalgh, T., Thorne, S. and Malterud, K. (2018) Time to challenge the spurious hierarchy of systematic over narrative reviews? *European Journal of Clinical Investigation* 48: 6.

Hariton, E. and Locascio, J.J. (2018) Randomised controlled trials – the gold standard for effectiveness research: Study design: Randomised controlled trials. *BJOG* 125 (13): 1716.

HCPC (Health and Care Professionals Council) (n.d.) Regulating health and care professionals. Available at https://www.hcpc-uk.org/?msclkid=24f42c24bb0b11ec9c26cffdb77d887e (accessed 29 March 2023).

Higgins, J.P.T., Thomas, J., Chandler, J., et al. (eds) (2022) *Cochrane Handbook for Systematic Reviews of Interventions version 6.3* (updated February 2022). Cochrane, 2022. Available at www.training.cochrane.org/handbook.

Ipsos MORI Social Research Institute (2019) *Evaluation of Revalidation for Nurses and Midwives: Year Three Report*. London: Ipsos. Available at ipsos-mori-revalidation-evaluation-report-year-3.pdf (nmc.org.uk) (accessed 24 May 2023).

Khan, K.S. and Zamora, J. (2022) *Systematic Reviews to Support Evidence-Based Medicine: How to Appraise, Conduct and Publish Reviews*, 3rd edn. London: Royal Society of Medicine Press.

Kumah, E.A., McSherry, R., Bettany-Saltikov, J. and Van Schaik, P. (2022) Evidence-informed practice: Simplifying and applying the concept for nursing students and academics. *British Journal of Nursing* 24;31 (6): 322–330.

Kunzler, M.M., Chmitorz, A., Röthke, N. et al. (2022) Interventions to foster resilience in nursing staff: A systematic review and meta-analyses of pre-pandemic evidence. *International Journal of Nursing Studies* 134: 1–28.

Law, M. and Baum, C. (1998) Evidence-based occupational therapy. *Canadian Journal of Occupational Therapy* 65 (3): 131–135.

Maung Htay, M. and Whitehead, D. (2021) The effectiveness of the role of advanced nurse practitioners compared to physician-led or usual care: A systematic review. *International Journal of Nursing Studies Advances* 3: 100034.

Muir Gray, J.A. (1997) *Evidence-Based Healthcare: How to Make Health Policy and Management Decisions*. London: Churchill Livingstone.

NIHR (National Institute for Health and Care Research) (2022) Glossary NIHR. Available at https://www.nihr.ac.uk/glossary/?letter=S&postcategory=-1 (accessed 9 November 2022).

NMC (Nursing and Midwifery Council) (n.d.) *The Code: Professional Standards of Practice and Behaviour for Nurses, Midwives and Nursing Associates*. Available at https://www.nmc.org.uk/globalassets/sitedocuments/nmc-publications/nmc-code.pdf (accessed 29 March 2023).

Pauling, L. (1974) Are recommended daily allowances for vitamin C adequate? *Proceedings of the National Academy of Sciences of the United States of America* 71 (11): 4442–4446.

Petticrew, M. and Roberts, II. (2006) *Systematic Reviews in the Social Sciences: A Practical Guide*. Oxford: Blackwell.

Purssell, E. and McCrae, N. (2020) *How to Perform a Systematic Literature Review: A Guide for Healthcare Researchers, Practitioners and Students*. Cham: Springer.

Rycroft-Malone, J., Seers, K., Titchen, A., Harvey, G., Kitson, A. and McCormack, B. (2004) What counts as evidence in evidence-based practice? *Journal of Advanced Nursing* 47: 81–90.

Sackett, D.L., Rosenberg, W.M., Gray, J.A., Haynes, R.B. and Richardson, W.S. (1996) Evidence based medicine: What it is and what it isn't. *British Medical Journal* 312 (7023): 71–72.

Santos, W.M.D., Secoli, S.R. and Püschel, V.A.A. (2018) The Joanna Briggs Institute approach for systematic reviews. *Rev Lat Am Enfermagem* 14 (26): e3074.

Tse, S., Lloyd, C., Penman, M., King, R. and Bassett, H. (2004) Evidence-based practice and rehabilitation: Occupational therapy in Australia and New Zealand experiences. *International Journal of Rehabilitation Research* 27 (4): 269–274.

Walker, K.J. and Terry, M.L. (2021) Factors influencing nurses' engagement with CPD activities: A systematic review. *British Journal of Nursing* 30 (1): 1–5.

Whitehead, B., Owen, P., Holmes, D. et al. (2013) Supporting newly qualified nurses in the UK: A systematic literature review. *Nurse Education Today* 33 (4): 370–377.

Wikipedia (2023) Archine Cochrane. Available at https://en.wikipedia.org/wiki/Archie_Cochrane (accessed 22 March 2023).

Youngblut, J.M. and Brooten, D. (2001) Evidence-based nursing practice: Why is it important? *AACN Clinical Issues: Advanced Practice in Acute and Critical Care* 12 (4): 468–476.

2

Asking an answerable and focused systematic review question

Overview

- Background work and preparation
- Selecting a topic area for your systematic review
- Narrowing the topic area to a specific, answerable systematic review question
- Using background or foreground questions: What is the difference?
- Factors to consider when asking an answerable and focused systematic review question
- Developing your systematic review question further
- Relating your systematic review question to the research design: What types of study designs should you look for to answer your systematic review question?
- Matching a specific research or review question to an appropriate research design

©123vector/123RF
Preparation is the Key

Background work and preparation

Some practical issues must be considered before work begins. It is important to make sure your project is actually feasible in terms of topic (not explored before), time, cost and so forth. It is also important to access the library either in person or online, to start looking at the top tips and early groundwork provided in Box 2.1. We would recommend you consider buying a notebook specifically for recording action points surrounding the systematic review (see Figure 2.1).

Box 2.1   Practical tips and early groundwork

- Go to the library.
- Ask colleagues about your topic and discuss it with them (importance, relevance, practical, doable, i.e. why and to whom is this important, what is it about, what are the potential benefits?).
- Where possible, create a systematic review team or team up with a group already doing a project in the area (this helps with sharing the workload and reviewing systems and processes).
- Consult patients/carers/members of the community who are affected by the areas to seek their opinions surrounding the need for the systematic review.
- It is really important to have patients' involvement and representation on the systematic review group.

A notebook helps you to:

- keep a record of progress
- keep ideas, appointments, outcomes of meetings all in one place
- make notes about different aspects of the study for example outcomes, themes, etc.
- keep useful newspaper articles as well as scientific papers
- reflect and record eureka moments and useful references.

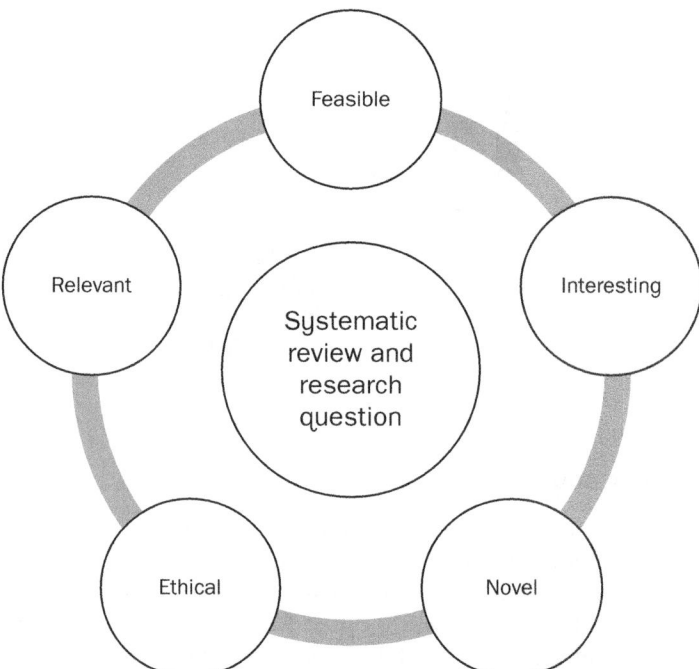

Figure 2.1 The FINER approach, adapted from Hulley et al. (2007).

Practical Tip

Having all this information together in one place makes the writing up of the project much easier at the end. Other things to consider when deciding on a systematic review question are the points outlined in Hulley et al.'s (2007) FINER approach.

The FINER approach

The FINER approach was developed by Professor Stephen Brian Hulley MD, MPH Professor and Chair, Department of Epidemiology and Biostatistics Director, Clinical and Translational Sciences Training Program University of California, San Francisco, and colleagues. The approach aims at building and highlighting the fundamental points of an appropriate academic study (Hulley et al. 2007). FINER (**F**easible, **I**nteresting, **N**ovel, **E**thical and **R**elevant) is a mnemonic system encompassing five characteristics to consider when developing your systematic review question (Figure 2.1).

Depicting the FINER approach in brief

The following are criteria to consider using when developing a systematic review question:

- **Feasible:** It is important that the student or researcher has an appreciation of research methodology to answer their proposed systematic review and/or research question. Novice systematic literature reviewers need to consider the resources, time and costs required to access databases, search for and examine the literature, critique the papers and write up the systematic review. You may also require the support of IT experts too, for example a statistician to conduct the meta-analysis and a librarian to support you in undertaking the searches. These are important to complete the systematic review to a high standard.
- **Interesting:** Keep in mind that your peers will be reviewing the title, protocol and final publication of your systematic review. Therefore, it is imperative to ensure your question is both interesting and contemporary to your profession. Ideally select a topic that is of a great interest to *you, your peers as well as patients and the public*. In our opinion, your research may be more effective if it engages with individuals who are both enthusiastic and ambitious.
- **Novel:** A systematic review can provide new insights and different perspectives, or identify changes to policy and practice in the field of study you are investigating, enabling you to confirm or refute existing research or practice. It is important that you are familiar with the previous and current literature of your field of expertise. Following this approach will help you, with your contribution, to improve 'the current body of evidence and debate around the topic area' (Hulley et al. 2007: 21–22).
- **Ethical:** The topic you select may be in an area for which approval by an ethical review board or authority is required. It is worth checking with the chair of your local university or other ethics committee prior to starting your systematic review.

- **Relevant:** Students or researchers usually choose topics related to their profession as well as the public's and patients' interest. Topics that are reproducible, applicable and important to patients and professionals may sometimes lead to visible changes in health and care services.

We recommend that you try and mitigate any potential challenges surrounding your systematic review. This will need to start at the outset, when choosing a well-structured topic. Applying the FINER approach to support the development of your systematic review and/or research question (as originally intended by Hulley et al. 2007) guides you through a series of questions supporting you to produce a quality answerable question that can only serve you in conducting and producing an outstanding systematic review.

Selecting a topic area for your systematic review

The first step towards undertaking your systematic review is to select a topic area. The specific topic area you select may arise from a number of different triggers.

If you are a nursing student, your interest in a topic may result from a lecture or module on a nursing condition that was covered in your undergraduate classes or a nursing problem that you or a patient and/or relative have experienced. The topic area may also arise from a contemporary issue highlighted in the media, such as reports on the latest research studies conducted, on falls or pressure sore prevention or on nursing interventions associated with keeping patients safe, for example ensuring they are well nourished as opposed to malnourished and avoiding medication errors.

If you are a practising nurse, it is likely that the topic area you choose will be related to your professional practice, clinical working or teaching and learning environment. It could also be an issue related to the Nursing and Midwifery Council (NMC) or a national initiative (see Box 2.2). Whatever your role and responsibility, it is

---

Box 2.2   Key points to remember when choosing a systematic review topic area

When choosing a systematic review topic area, you will need to identify:

- an area you are interested in related to your practice
- a question that you would like to know the answer to
- why the question is interesting and worth investigating
- issues relating to the question
- what you will gain by investigating the question
- what your profession and other professions will gain
- the rationale for asking the question
- the use of having the answer, i.e. 'So what?'
- the lack of knowledge in the area – this means you need to show the gap in the literature
- an awareness of how the review question may improve safety, quality, health and practice.

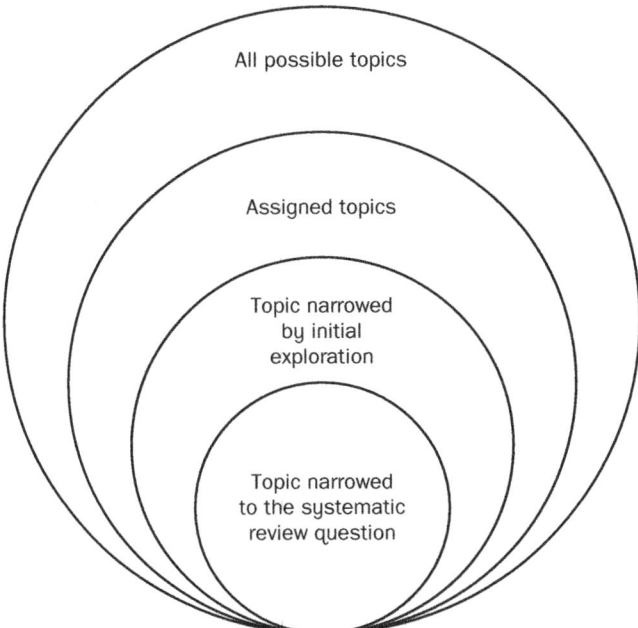

All possible topics

Assigned topics

Topic narrowed
by initial
exploration

Topic narrowed
to the systematic
review question

Figure 2.2 Selecting and focusing your topic area.

important that when selecting your review topic area, you take into account a number
of key points by working from the broad towards the specific (Figure 2.2).

> **Practical Tip**
>
> To identify an appropriate review question, try focusing on an aspect of nursing
> practice that may arise from a thank-you letter, an incident, an event and/or
> aspects of the clinical environment or professional practice that are highly topical
> and recurring situations. You may also consider those topics or issues that are reg-
> ularly discussed and debated in multidisciplinary team and/or clinical meetings.

Narrowing the topic area to a specific, answerable review question

Once you have selected your review topic area, the next step is to narrow this down to
a systematic review question. This process is similar to a funnel or an inverted triangle
(see Figure 2.3), where the wide base of the funnel represents the review topic and the
narrow peak at the other end represents the specific review question.

To illustrate the above, a student nurse who is interested in spinal deformities
might select spinal deformities as the topic area. One specific question arising from
this specific topic could be related to 'the effectiveness of braces for treating patients
with scoliosis'. Here the student nurse has narrowed the topic area by specifying both
the treatment (braces) as well as the type of spinal deformity (scoliosis).

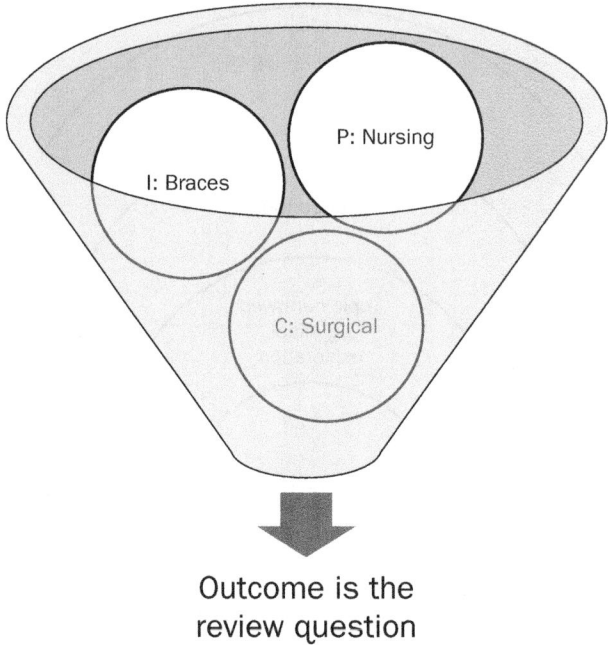

Figure 2.3 Deriving the review question from the topic area.

Another registered nurse working in the accident and emergency (A&E) department may be interested in witnessed resuscitation (where family members are present during resuscitation attempts), as they have participated in a number of these procedures during routine practice. 'Witnessed resuscitation' would then be the general topic area and a possible review question arising from this area could be 'What are the views of qualified nurses regarding witnessed resuscitation in the A&E department?' Here the registered nurse has narrowed the topic area to a review question by specifying that the views of qualified nurses on this topic will be the focus. Furthermore, this will be restricting the review to qualified nurses working in the A&E department.

You may be wondering 'How do you actually derive the question from the topic?' The way to do this is to ask a series of questions that will narrow the topic down. To illustrate how this is done, we will use a hypothetical case study of a spinal nurse called Tamara (Box 2.3). Once you have read the case study you can try to narrow down your own topic area to a systematic review question using the template provided in Box 2.4.

Template to help you develop your systematic review question from your review topic area

Box 2.4 contains a template, adapted from the works of Bailey (1997) and Hissong et al. (2015), that you can use to help focus your own systematic review question. Once you have decided on a specific problem area and review question, the next step is to refine and break down the systematic review question and make it as comprehensive

---

𝕋 Box 2.3 Case study: Tamara, a spinal nurse

Tamara is a spinal nurse working in a new spinal unit. As part of her role in the spinal deformity department she takes care of many teenagers who suddenly develop a spinal deformity when they reach their teens, a condition known as adolescent idiopathic (unknown cause) scoliosis (AIS). Before developing this deformity, when they were children, their spines were normal. The cause for this is not yet known, so the treatment concentrates on the symptoms. One of the treatments that Tamara is involved in is scoliosis-specific exercises and braces to treat the spinal curvatures, to try to reduce these curvatures and rib prominence. These patients may have several psychological issues, such as low self-esteem and self-image as well as occasional pain. Tamara would like to conduct a systematic review to find the evidence underpinning the *effectiveness of the practice of braces and scoliosis-specific exercises.* This is an example of a systematic review question.

Box 2.4 Focusing the review question from the topic area (adapted from Bailey 1995; Hissong et al. 2015)

1. Write down the original systematic review question.
2. State the general topic area of your project. Is there something wrong with it?
3. What is the specific problem you plan to address? Is there something wrong with it?
4. Does something need attention?
5. Who is the individual, group or community that will engage in the project?
6. Is something missing? (This is where the gap in the literature may be found.)
7. Do old ideas need to be revisited?
8. Practise writing your review question several different ways to expand or limit the options of your review.
9. Give at least three reasons why your review agenda is important and valid to you, your society and your profession. Why is your study important?
10. What is the benefit of this study? Who would benefit from the review?
11. What might happen if the review is not done?
12. Write a significance statement.
13. State what you hope to accomplish regarding the review that you are going to engage in.
14. What do you hope to accomplish regarding the problem by carrying out your review?
15. Who are the individuals, groups or community members this research will impact in a beneficial way?
16. Will you change something?
17. Will you understand something?
18. Will you interpret something differently?

and specific as possible. To do this you will need to consider the different categories of systematic review questions: not only are there background and foreground questions, but there are also different types of foreground questions. Your systematic review will differ based on whether you are investigating the effectiveness of a treatment programme, seeking to prevent a condition occurring, diagnosing a medical problem, looking at the cause or prognosis of a specific condition or disease, or exploring patients', users' or nurses' perceptions and experiences.

Box 2.5 provides a completed version of the template in Box 2.4.

Box 2.5   An example of how to focus the review question from the topic area (adapted from Bailey 1995; Hissong et al. 2015)

1. Write down the original review question:

What are the effects of braces and scoliosis-specific exercises for teenagers with AIS?

2. State the general topic area of your project. Is there something wrong with it?

Possible answer: The general area of the project is spinal deformities. This is too vague, as we need to know the specific pathology, the population, intervention and outcome measures to be used.

3. What is the specific problem you plan to address? Is there something wrong with it?

The specific problem I plan to address is the management of young teenagers using a brace and scoliosis exercises to treat the scoliosis deformity. In this version it is stated too vaguely.

4. Does something need attention?

Yes. It is currently unclear whether braces and/or scoliosis exercises are effective and for which curve size.

5. Who is the individual, group or community that will engage in the project?

Patients with AIS, researchers, clinicians, parents and family members of service users.

6. Is something missing? (This is where the gap in the literature may be found.)

Yes, historically teenagers with AIS were not always afforded the opportunity to receive braces and physiotherapeutic scoliosis-specific exercises (PSSE).

7. Do old ideas need to be revisited?

Yes. Currently the scoliosis pathway is mainly surgical. It is only recently beginning to consider non-surgical interventions.

8. Practise writing your review question several different ways to expand or limit the options of your review.

- For patients with AIS, which intervention is best? This is a very open question and not all the PICOT (population, intervention, comparative intervention or group, outcome and type of study) elements are included.

- For patients with AIS, which intervention is best: surgical or non-surgical treatment? Again this question is more limited and the outcomes are still not included.
- What are the effects on rib-hump, spinal curvature and psychological factors of non-surgical and surgical treatment of adolescents with idiopathic scoliosis who have moderate to severe curves?

9. Give at least three reasons why your review agenda is important and valid to you, your society and your profession. Why is your study important?

- It is important and valid to me as a researcher, as my research is in this area of study.
- My society: Scoliosis patients will benefit from non-invasive treatment, and this may improve their quality of life.
- My profession: If the review finds that conservative treatment is more effective than non-surgical treatment, it may be used more in the UK. This will possibly save young children from having to undergo big operations.
- Why is your review important? As above. Also, this will also possibly save the NHS a lot of money and save many young people from having major surgery.
- What can happen that will be beneficial if the review is done? As above.

10. What is the benefit of this study? Who would benefit from the review?

The patients and their families will benefit as well as clinicians involved in their treatment. Researchers and other stakeholders will also benefit.

11. What might happen if the review is not done?

If the review is not done and published, patients will continue to be treated as they always have. This means 'watching the curve' till the scoliosis angle is 50 degrees or more and then surgery as a first treatment choice.

12. Write a significance statement.

(The significance is the importance of your particular study and what this will do to help the larger problem. It is the 'So what?' part of the study.) The study is of great importance to young people who develop AIS and their families for the first time in the NHS as it will allow them to have the choice of having PSSE when their curves are small. This means they may be able to possible avoid braces which are very uncomfortable and well as surgery together with any potential complications. It also means that the patients will be allowed to get treated sooner with the hopes of preventing the progression of the curve.

13. State what you hope to accomplish regarding the review that you are going to engage in.

We hope to eventually change the scoliosis pathway to start with non-invasive treatment (braces and exercises) rather than surgery.

14. What do you hope to accomplish regarding the problem by carrying out your review?

As above.

15. Who are the individuals, groups or community members this research will impact in a beneficial way?

The service users as well as all the healthcare professionals who treat them, i.e. specialist scoliosis physiotherapists, orthotists, surgeons.

16. Will you change something?

Yes. Ideally scoliosis school screening can be initiated to identify students with small curves who can be treated with PSSE. These could then be referred to a scoliosis specialist physiotherapist who is trained in the assessment and treatment of this problem. If the curve continures to grow then the patients could be referred onto the scoliosis surgeon.

17. Will you understand something?

Yes. We will know that conservative treatment is effective for the treatment of small curves.

18. Will you interpret something differently?

Yes. It will mean that clinical practice will need to change.

Practical Tip

We recommend reading at least 10 abstracts on a closely related topic. The abstracts generally focus on the background, purpose and significance of the research study and can be invaluable in helping you focus on your own systematic review. Abstracts are valuable as they are a good way of helping you understand what was done in a primary research study. Reviewing abstracts is an excellent way in helping you understand what should be included to produce a good abstract of your own.

Using background or foreground questions: What is the difference?

Background questions refer to general nursing questions about a patient. These can be systematic review questions about a nursing/medical condition, such as: What causes the condition? How is it treated? Is it an issue related to nursing intervention and/or the clinical environmental? Are patient safety and the quality of care an issue? The answers to these questions can be found in background sources such as textbooks or narrative reviews, which give an *overview* of the topic area.

Foreground questions answer a *specific* question about a specific topic. Foreground sources can be divided into primary sources such as original research articles published in peer-reviewed journals and secondary sources such as systematic reviews of the topic and synopses and reviews of individual studies. Secondary sources are one step removed from the original research. Table 2.1 gives some

Table 2.1 The types of studies in foreground sources

Primary sources – original research	Secondary sources – reviews of original research
Experimental studies (an intervention is made) • Randomized controlled trial (RCT) • Controlled trials **Observational studies** (no intervention is done, no variables are manipulated) • Cohort studies • Case-control studies • Case reports/case studies **Qualitative research studies** • Phenomenological, ethnographic or grounded theory studies	• Systematic reviews • Systematic reviews with a meta-analysis • Practice and policy guidelines • Decision analysis • Consensus reports • Editorial, commentary

examples of primary and secondary sources. The various concepts listed in the table are explained in this chapter.

Building the systematic review question

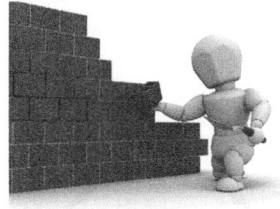

©kjpargeter/123RF

Factors to consider when asking an answerable and focused systematic review question

Blaikie (2007) suggests that the use of systematic review questions is a neglected aspect in the design and conduct of research and that formulating a systematic review and/or 'research question is the most critical and perhaps the most difficult part of any research [systematic review] design' (Blaikie 2007: 6). The formulation of the systematic review question is crucial because the question underpins all the aspects of the systematic review methodology: every single step of the systematic review is determined by the focused systematic review question. The function of a systematic review question can be summed up as in the box that follows.

Practical Tip

Developing a focused question: Why do we need this?

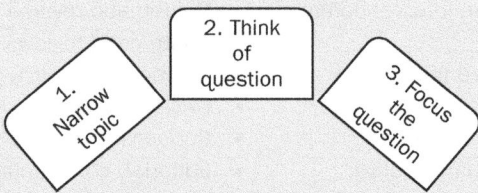

Having a clear, focused and answerable systematic review question has a number of benefits:

- It clarifies the problem in your own mind.
- It helps to identify the types of evidence you will need to answer the systematic review question.
- It helps to identify the key terms to answer your systematic review question.
- It will therefore lead to more relevant information being found in your search(es).
- It will help identify your population, intervention, comparative group and outcomes as well as the type of study designs (explored in detail later in this chapter).

Asking open questions, not closed ones

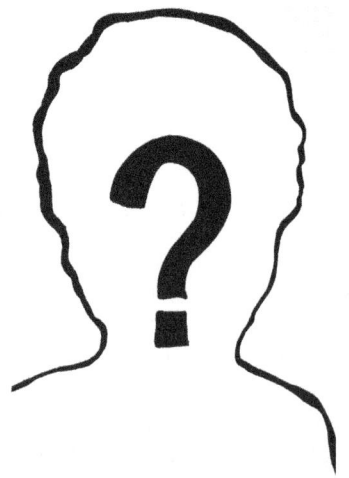

When formulating a systematic review question, it is important to ensure that you *ask an open question and not make a statement*. For example, rather than making a statement saying, 'Braces improve the spinal curvatures of patients with scoliosis', as a novice student might, it would be preferable to ask the systematic review question, 'What effect do spinal braces have on patients with spinal curvatures?' In the first example you are making an assumption that braces will actually improve the back when they might not, and they may even make the back worse. In this example you are making a statement and not asking a question. The first example is similar to a closed question and could introduce some bias (or errors).

The second example is an open question and less biased. Asking this type of question will allow you to find research papers that discuss all the different effects of braces, both positive and negative.

Tips on the actual wording of the systematic review question

To help you to write a good, answerable systematic review question it is important to consider how you word a question: it is best *to avoid questions that can be answered with a simple yes or no*. For example, the question 'Do braces have an effect on the spinal curvatures of patients with spinal deformities?' can easily be answered with a yes or a no, whereas 'What effect do spinal braces have on patients with spinal curvatures?' encourages more discussion and is more open and unbiased.

Table 2.2 lists a number of different review questions to help you determine what sort of evidence you are looking for within the primary research papers that you will select to answer your review question. One way to facilitate the development of your systematic review question is to determine what kind of question you are asking (Anastasiadis et al. 2015). The next step will be to match the systematic review question to the specific systematic review design. From there you can work out what kind of evidence you will need.

The main types of systematic review questions

Some examples from practice can be found below:

1 **Examples of treatment/therapy questions**
    - What are the effects of braces on patients with spinal deformities?
    - How effective are anti-depressive medications for anxiety and depression?
    - How effective are pressure-relieving mattresses at avoiding pressure sores?
    - How effective are hip protectors at avoiding fractures of the femur?
2 **Examples of prevention questions**
    - For patients of 70 years and older, how effective is the use of the influenza vaccine at preventing flu as compared with patients who have not received the vaccine?
    - How effective is school screening for scoliosis in reducing the risk of future surgery in patients with scoliosis?
    - How effective is intentional rounding in improving the quality of the patient experience?

Table 2.2 Main types of research questions

	Type	Description	Illustration
1	**Treatment/therapy** ©enrarokudou/123RF	Which treatment is most effective? Does it do more good than harm?	Is the use of dressing A better than dressing B in the treatment of venous leg ulcers?
2	**Prevention** ©iuphotos/123RF	How can the risk of disease be reduced?	Do increasing levels of obesity increase the risk of developing diabetes?
3	**Diagnosis** ©krasimiranevenova/123RF	How should one select and interpret diagnostic tests?	Is having an X-ray as effective as having a computerized tomography (CT) scan for diagnosing a brain tumour?
4	**Prognosis** ©iuphotos/123RF	How can one anticipate the likely course of the disease?	Are babies who are bottle fed more likely to be obese once they reach adulthood, compared with babies who are breastfed?
5	**Causation (cause)** ©artursz/123RF	What are the risk factors for developing certain conditions?	Does exposure to parental alcohol during pregnancy increase the risk of foetal alcohol syndrome in newborn babies?
6	**Experiences or perceptions**	How do people feel about this treatment or disease?	How do patients experience life with a venous leg ulcer ?

3   **Examples of diagnosis questions**
- In patients with suspected anorexia nervosa, what is the accuracy of a new scale compared with the 'gold standard', previously validated instrument?
- In patients with suspected scoliosis (spinal curvature), what is the accuracy of a new non-invasive surface topography scanning device as compared with X-rays?

4   **Examples of prognosis questions**
- How much more likely are babies who are bottle fed to catch colds than babies who are breastfed?
- How much more likely are workers with musculoskeletal disorders to take sick leave as compared with workers diagnosed with stress?
- How much more likely are children who are screened for scoliosis to have surgery than children who are not screened?

5   **Examples of causation questions**
- For healthy post-menopausal patients on hormone replacement therapy (HRT), what are the increased risks for developing breast cancer?
- In women taking oral contraceptives, is there an association between their use and breast cancer?
- Does having a parent with a spinal deformity increase the risk of the child developing scoliosis once they reach puberty?

6   **Examples of questions related to patients' experiences/perspectives**
- What are teenagers' experiences of living with a spinal brace?
- How do older patients experience life with cancer?
- What are student nurses' experiences of life as first-year university students?

Developing your systematic review question further: A framework for developing a focused question

To search effectively, the systematic review question that you are trying to answer needs identifying. To do this, it needs separating into several different parts. So, what are these parts?

- P stands for population (the group you are interested in reviewing).
- I is for intervention and E is for exposure (the type of treatment, care provided, or experience of illness/disease).
- C is for comparative group or intervention (generally comparing a new treatment against the usual standard of treatment).
- O is for outcomes (the benefits or not of what are you measuring).
- T is for type of study design that you are interested in reviewing.

The acronym for this is PICOT, which stands for population, intervention, comparative group or intervention, outcome and type of study. PICOT is designed mainly for questions of therapeutic interventions (Khan and Zamora 2022). Another useful acronym is PEOT, which stands for patient, exposure, outcome and type of study. PEOT is used most frequently for qualitative questions (Khan and Zamora 2022).

Practical Tip

Having identified the relevant literature, it is important to separate the question into several different yet significant parts. These are:

1. P=population

2. I=intervention

3. C=comparative group

4. O=Outcomes

5. T=type of study design

Question formulation

If you have followed all of the steps above, you should by now have a tentative systematic review question. To search for all the relevant papers on the topic, it is *essential* that your question is both *comprehensive* and *specific*. It should include *only one question* and not two or three questions.

A good way to identify the different parts of your question for PICOT formats is to make a table containing five rows, one for each letter of the acronym. A well-framed review question will have at least five elements. For your own question, think about and write down one PICOT and one PEOT question.

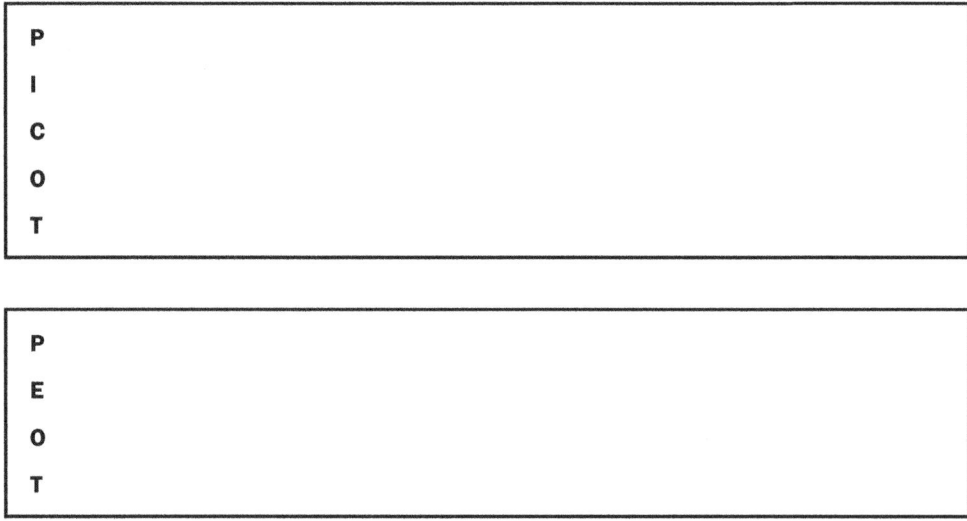

P
I
C
O
T

P
E
O
T

Table 2.3 shows what type of information to include in each of the sections for PICOT questions. Table 2.4 shows some completed examples. For qualitative questions that use the PEOT format you will need to create a table containing four rows. Table 2.5 shows you what to include in each section.

Table 2.3 Component parts to consider when asking clear, focused review questions

P Population and their diagnosis	Here you need to state the clinical diagnosis or disease and the age, gender and any other relevant factors related to the population you would like to include. The population group needs to be specified regardless of which type of question you are considering.
I or E Intervention or exposure	If you are planning to evaluate a specific intervention, you will need to state the type of intervention that you are seeking to evaluate, such as the type of drug and any specifics related to it, like dosage and other relevant factors. If you are not looking at an intervention but are considering a specific 'exposure' (this term is used loosely), such as 'witnessed resuscitation' or 'domestic violence', you should use the E as in the PEOT acronym instead of the PICOT acronym. The exposure component can also be regarded as an 'issue' that the patients or the population you are considering including in your review have undergone.
C Comparative intervention	In a therapeutic question you will usually have a comparator (even if it is standard care). It is also possible to look at interventions without including a comparative intervention. For qualitative review questions or those involving a specific exposure or issue, this component is usually left out.
O Outcomes or themes	When writing down your outcomes, you need to consider the factors or issues you are looking for or measuring. For example, are you looking for any improvements in pain or mobility, or any other outcomes? With qualitative studies these will usually be the patients' and/or the nurse 'healthcare worker' experiences.
T Type of study design	It is important to include the research design in your review question for a number of reasons. It helps other researchers or students find a study containing a specific design, e.g. an RCT or phenomenological study. It helps librarians catalogue the review. It also clarifies to readers straight away what type of research design your review is about.

In Tables 2.4 and 2.5 you can find some examples of using both the PICOT and the PEOT acronyms to formulate your own questions. The PICOT questions are usually quantitative review questions and the PEOT ones are usually qualitative review questions.

Let's return to Tamara's question from the case study (Box 2.3 on p. 31). The structured question can be broken down into the component parts as defined by the PICOT framework as follows:

- In patients with adolescent idiopathic scoliosis (P)
- how effective is spinal bracing (I)
- as compared with observation (C)
- at reducing spinal curvature, rib hump and psychological problems (O)?
- Cohort studies (T)

Table 2.4 Examples of using PICOT to ask clear quantitative questions

	Example 1	*Example 2*	*Example 3*	*Example 4*
P Population and their problems	In patients with acute asthma	In children with a spinal deformity	In children with a fever	Among family members of patients with mental health problems
I Intervention or issue	How effective are antibiotics?	How effective is bracing?	How effective is paracetamol?	How effective is listening to tranquil music or recorded comedy routines?
C Comparative intervention	As compared with standard care	As compared with observation	As compared with ibuprofen	As compared with standard care (none)
O Outcomes or themes	At reducing sputum production and coughing	At reducing the scoliosis curvature	At reducing fever and infection	In reducing reported anxiety
T Type of study	Cohort RCT	Cohort RCT	Ethnography or cohort RCT, controlled clinical trial (CCT)	RCT CCT

Table 2.5 Examples of using PEOT to ask clear qualitative questions

	Example 1	*Example 2*	*Example 3*	*Example 4*
P Population and their problems	Teenagers with a spinal deformity	Older patients with cancer	Student nurses in their first year at university	Family members of patients with mental health problems
E Exposure	Having a spinal deformity	Having cancer	Studying to be a nurse at university and in their first year	Having a family member with a mental health issue
O Outcomes or themes	The patients' views	The patients' views	The students' views	The patients' views
T Type of study design	Phenomenology	Phenomenology or ethnography	Ethnography or grounded theory	Phenomenology

Table 2.6 Separating the component parts of Tamara's question using the PICOT method

P	I	C	O	T
Patients with AIS	spinal bracing …	… as compared with other treatments …	… at reducing spinal curvature, rib hump and psychological problems?	RCT CCT

Table 2.7 Christine's question broken down using the PEOT method

P	E	O	T
Patients with AIS	Having scoliosis and wearing a brace	Lived experiences of having scoliosis and wearing a brace	Phenomenological

Table 2.6 shows how to separate the component parts of Tamara's question using the PICOT method.

Tamara's nursing colleague Christine, who works in the same spinal unit, is more interested in the patients' views. Christine's question is: 'What are the lived experiences of patients with AIS of having scoliosis and wearing a brace?' Table 2.7 shows how Christine's question would be separated into its component parts using the PEOT acronym.

Practice session 2.1

A well-framed research question will have four or five elements. (However, most questions have at least five parts.) Now that we have seen how to split different types of questions into their component parts, why don't you try to split your own question? Use the templates provided in Boxes 2.6 and 2.7 to divide your intervention or exposure question into PICOT or PEOT. If your question has more than one population group, adapt the template as appropriate.

Box 2.6 Template for splitting a quantitative intervention question into PICOT component parts

P	I	C	O	T

Box 2.7 Template for splitting a qualitative experience question into PEOT component parts

P	E	O	T

Examples of review questions with commentary

Practice session 2.2

Read the review questions and commentary below and see if you can identify all the PICOT or PEOT elements for each one, noting if any of the elements are missing.

Example review question 1

Question: 'A comparison of surgical and conservative management in adults in terms of functional outcome, union rates and post-operative complications.'

Commentary:

The above review question is a statement and not a question.

P: The population in this example is described as 'adults'. However, this is much too vague. The population needs to be more specific and include the disease or medical condition as well as the severity of the disease. You also need to specify the type of adults you are referring to. Do these adults have some health condition?

I: We can also see that the outcomes relate to union rates, functional outcomes and post-op complications. This suggests that these adults have a fracture. The location is not identified. The 'question' also states conservative and surgical management. However, which ones specifically? There are several different conservative and operative treatment interventions. So, the question needs to specify exactly what the intervention is, for example whether it is operative or non-operative treatment that these adults are undergoing.

O: Furthermore, the outcomes are very vague. Which outcomes exactly and how will these outcomes be measured? So, the functional outcome (e.g. mobility, union rates) of the arm or leg? The union rates in the leg take much more time to heal. Also, which specific operative complications are we talking about?

T: The type of design is omitted. You could consider including RCTs, CCTs or experiment-type studies. Alternatively, you could explore patient and/or staff experiences of undergoing this type of intervention.

The question above could be rewritten as follows:

What are the operative (hip surgery) and non-operative (traction) treatment outcomes in older adult patients (>70 years old) with a hip fracture in terms of mobility, gait and post-op complications six weeks (short term) and one year (long term) after surgery?

So, what have we changed? We have:

- changed the statement to a review question
- specified the surgical and non-surgical interventions
- identified exactly what the outcomes are, as well as when the outcomes will be measured
- articulated who the population will be: adults over 70 years old who have had a hip fracture.

A final note: Before you settle on your specific question, it is very important to know what each treatment entails and to make sure that they are both appropriate and relevant for the chronic disease you select. In essence, the question or statement above needs to be built up again from the beginning, apart from the intervention section.

Example review question 2

Question: 'Patient experiences of the use of complementary and alternative therapies (CAT) in patients with chronic disease.

Commentary:

The review question is a statement and not a review question. Let us explore the rationale for this in more detail. We use either the PICOT or PEOT to help reconstruct the review question. Before you settle on your final review question, it is important to know what the potential complementary and /or alternative therapies you are considering entail, and why you have chosen to look at these for the chronic disease you have selected. Is there sufficient evidence to corroborate or refute the potential claims?

In essence the review question needs to be refocused and developed from the beginning using either of the acronyms above. A possible approach may be to select two different types of CATs and either include both or compare them to each other, so you move from a statement to a review question. It is important to identify the nature and type of chronic disease you are considering for your review question.

Similarly, the inclusion of the words 'experiences' and 'perspectives' in the title suggests that this is a qualitative question. The term 'complementary and alternative therapies' is also vague. It is imperative to demonstrate how these potential interventions effect the chronic disease from progression or helps improve the patient's quality of life. For example, looking at the effectiveness of acupuncture for patients with type 2 diabetes in improving blood sugars and reducing pain attributed to peripheral neuropathy. You could even focus on health and well-being activities, such as walking, swimming and strength training.

P: The population in this example is described as patients with chronic disease. This is a broad term incorporating many different types of diseases, for example diabetes, high blood pressure, scoliosis, different types of cancer, and chronic obstructive pulmonary disease. It would help to include the age, gender and time in years.

I: The intervention in this example is acupuncture, but it could also have been reiki, tai chi, aromatherapy, etc.

C: For this review question you could consider comparing the effectiveness of acupuncture and/or another type of CAT. Alternatively, you could omit a comparator and just focus on one type of CAT.

O: Outcomes could be specifically targeted and include measurements such as blood sugar levels over time, pain scale readings and quality-of-life measures.

T: Type of study designs could be qualitative studies, such as phenomenological, ethnographic, grounded theory and action research.

The question above could, for example, be rewritten as follows:

What are the experiences of older adult patients (over 65 years) who have lived with type 2 diabetes for more than five years, following the use of acupuncture?: A qualitative systematic review.

Or

What are the experiences of older adult patients (over 65 years) who have lived with type 2 diabetes for more than five years, following the use of acupuncture and aromatherapy?: A qualitative systematic review.

So, what have we changed? We have:

- changed the statement to a review question
- identified the chronic disease (type 2 diabetes) and the length of time living with the disease
- specified the CAT interventions (either acupuncture alone and/or combined with aromatherapy)
- identified what the associated outcomes are (experiences)
- articulated the population (adults over 65 years old)
- identified the study design (qualitative).

As a final note: Before you finalize your review question, it is important to ensure that each element of the PICOT or the PEOT are articulated and check with someone else.

Relating your review question to the research design (T) of your chosen papers: What types of study designs should you look for to answer your research question?

Now that you have split your question into its component parts, the next step is to think about how your review question relates to the research design of the studies that you plan to include within your review. These will form the basis for answering your review question.

Why do we need to consider this? The above is important for several reasons:

- It allows you to focus your review question by targeting the specific primary research papers aligned to your review question. Secondary research papers cannot be included as the key papers within your review.

- Some authors of systematic reviews recommend the inclusion of the type of study design (T) of the proposed studies while still in the process of formulating your review question (Khan and Zamora 2022). So rather than using PICO or PEO you could adapt this to use PICOT or PEOT, where the T stands for the *type* of study or research design, as explained above.

- The type of research design can be thought of as the structure of the research study. It is a plan of how all the parts of the project fit together, including who the subjects are, what instruments were used (if any), how the study was conducted and analysed and, finally, how it is discussed.

Types of quantitative research designs

A number of common quantitative research designs are described in Figures 2.4 and 2.6.

Case report, case study, case series

A case report is a report of a treatment of an individual patient. Case reports are generally undertaken and reported when a patient of particular interest or with special or complex characteristics is treated by a nurse, doctor or other health and care professional. For example, you may come across a patient who has a condition that you have never seen or heard of before and you are uncertain what to do. A search for case series or case reports may reveal information that will help you treat your patient. When the first case of Creutzfeldt-Jakob disease (CJD, commonly known as mad cow disease) was treated, it would have been reported as a case study. When a few cases are reported, this becomes a case series. Figure 2.5 illustrates the design of a case report study, with the schematic for a case report and case series research design.

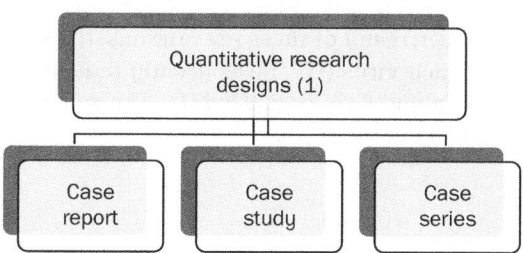

Figure 2.4 Three types of quantitative research designs.

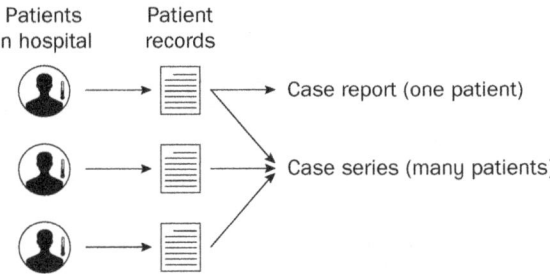

Figure 2.5 A schematic for a case report and case series.

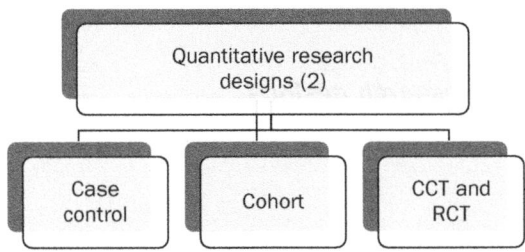

Figure 2.6 More quantitative research designs.

Case-control studies

Case-control studies are research studies in which patients who **already have** a specific condition are compared with people who do not. These studies rely on medical records and patient recall for data collection. In other words, they are retrospective studies (looking back) that can be undertaken quickly by documenting the patients' histories. A good example of this can be seen by considering the time during the acquired immune deficiency syndrome (AIDS) epidemic, when case-control studies identified not only risk groups such as homosexual men, intravenous drug users and blood transfusion recipients, but also risk factors, such as having multiple sexual partners and not using condoms. Based on such studies, blood banks restricted high-risk individuals from donating blood and educational programmes began to promote safer sexual behaviours. As a result of these precautions, the speed of transmission of the human immunodeficiency virus (HIV) was greatly reduced, even before the virus had been identified (Schulz and Grimes 2002: 431). The schematic for a case-control research design can be seen in Figure 2.7.

Cohort studies

Cohort studies are usually made up of a large population. The cohort study design follows patients who have a specific condition or who receive a particular treatment over time. These patients are compared with another group that has not been affected

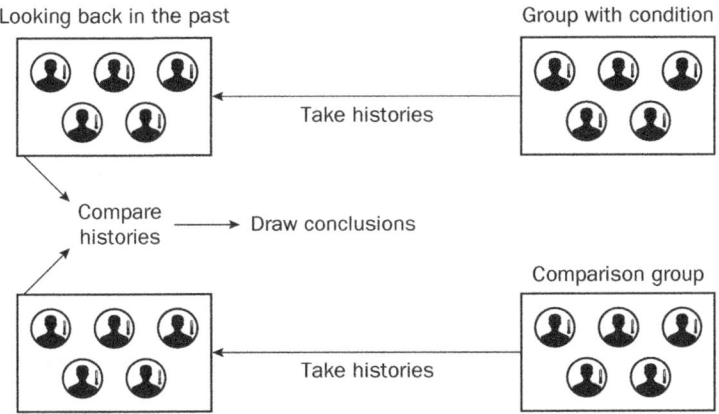

Figure 2.7 A schematic for a case-control research design.

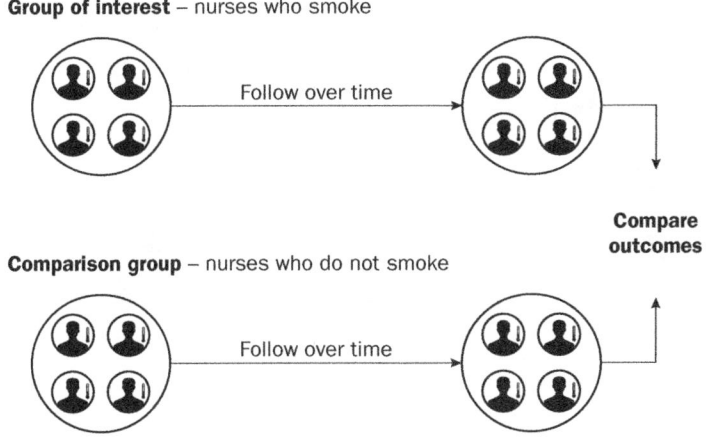

Figure 2.8 A schematic for a cohort research design.

by the condition or treatment. For example, you may be interested in the long-term effects of smoking on nurses. In a cohort study you would follow-up a group of nurses who smoke and a group who do not smoke and then compare their outcomes over time. One of the main problems with this type of research design is that they can take a very long time to conduct. If you started following both groups of nurses when they were in their twenties and measured the outcomes every 10 years until they retired, this would mean the study would take over 40 years to complete. The schematic for a cohort research design can be seen in Figure 2.8.

RCTs and CCTs

In RCTs the effect of treatments such as therapy, medication or programmes on real patients is studied. The methods they include are aimed at reducing the potential for bias and the patients may be randomly assigned into a treatment group and a control group. The control group have the same conditions as the treated group, but they are not given the treatment. This allows us to be certain that it was the treatment itself that had an effect on the patients and not anything else. A schematic for an RCT research design can be seen in Figure 2.9.

The CCT design is very similar to the RCT design, but there is no randomization of participants.

Systematic reviews

As discussed in Chapter 1, an extensive and systematic literature review is conducted that uses only studies with sound methodology. The studies are collected, reviewed and assessed, data are extracted and the results are summarized according to the pre-determined criteria of the review question (see Figure 2.10).

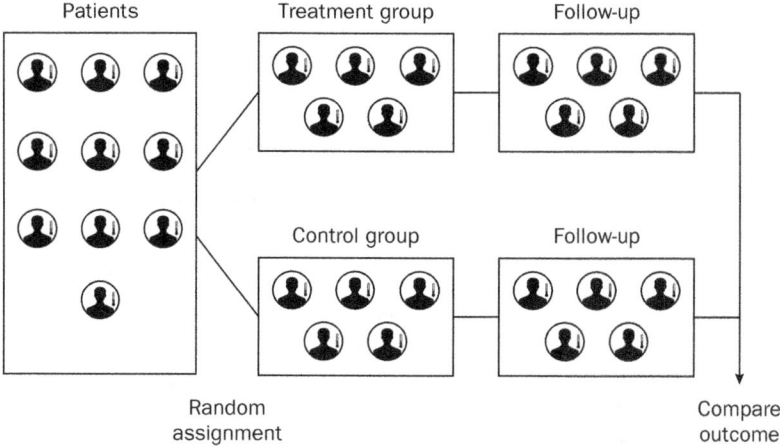

Figure 2.9 A schematic for an RCT research design.

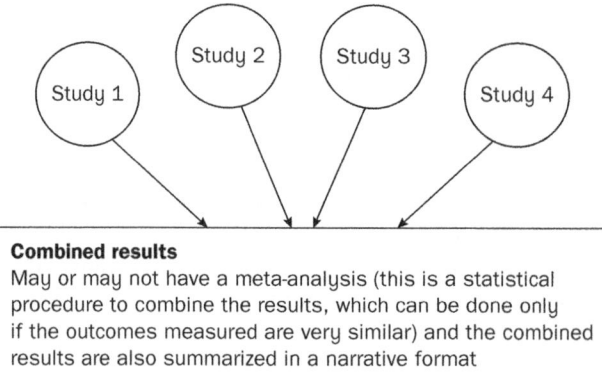

Figure 2.10 An illustration of how several studies can be combined to produce a definitive result.

Meta-analysis

In brief, a meta-analysis is a statistical procedure that is used in some systematic reviews. A meta-analysis examines a group of valid quantitative studies on a topic and combines the results using accepted statistical methodology to reach a consensus on the overall results. A meta-analysis can be used only on studies where the research papers included are similar and where the outcome measures of the included research papers are the same. Only a small proportion of systematic reviews include a meta-analysis. (Please refer to Chapter 13 for more details on how to conduct this.)

Types of qualitative research designs

The three most common types of qualitative research designs are described in Figure 2.11.

Phenomenological research design

When nurses apply a phenomenological research design, they are concerned with the lived experiences of people (Greene 1997). This could be the lived experiences of patients with a particular condition, the experiences of older nurses, or the experiences of nursing students while training in hospitals. For example, in Table 2.1 earlier in this chapter the patient could be asked what their experience of being a patient in an intensive care unit was like.

Ethnographic research design

You may be interested to know that the Stanford Ethnography Lab supports ethnographic and fieldwork research through offering graduate fellowships, workshops, seminars and collaborative opportunities (Stanford University n.d.). An ethnographic research design was originally used by anthropologists who went to live with native people in remote places to gain a deeper understanding of how they lived. According to Spradley (1979: 3), ethnography is 'the work of describing a culture' and the goal of ethnographic research is 'to understand another way of life from the native point of view'. Within nursing practice, the term 'native' is used loosely and could refer, for example, to different

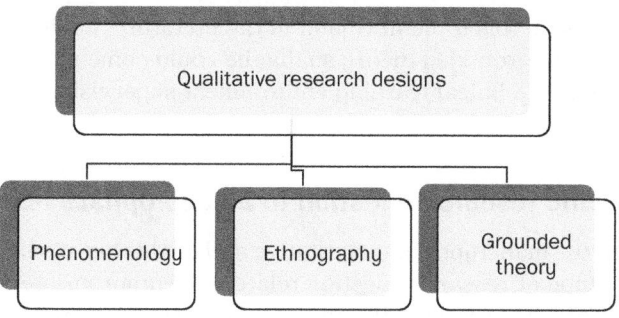

Figure 2.11 Three types of qualitative research designs.

nursing cultures that can be found within mental health nursing as compared with adult and paediatric nursing. Spradley (1979: iv) suggests that ethnography is a useful tool for 'understanding how other people see their experience'. He emphasizes, however, that 'rather than *studying people*, ethnography means *learning from people*' (Spradley 1979: 3, our emphases). If we apply this in a nursing context, we may be interested in learning from nurses who work in a specific culture or area, such as mental health nurses who work in prisons, nurses who work in an intensive care unit or nurses who work in palliative care, comparing similar roles internationally. Similarly, the research may focus on the lived experience of patients/carers who have stayed within these clinical environments and settings.

There have recently been advances in the development and application of online ethnography (also known as virtual ethnography or digital ethnography). This is a computer-based platform using various research approaches, utilizing and modifying ethnographic methods to explore different communities and cultures through various social media and interacting platforms. More information can be found in Pink et al (2015).

Grounded theory research design

The grounded theory research design was developed by Glaser and Strauss (1967). This method is used as both a qualitative research method and a method of data analysis. In grounded theory the researcher aims to develop a theory that can explain events and behaviours, making predictions and providing us with control over a situation. Grounded theory is a research method that operates almost in a reverse fashion from traditional research; at first it may appear to be contradictory to the scientific method (Noble and Mitchell 2016). Rather than beginning with a hypothesis, the first step is data collection, through a variety of methods. From the data collected, the key points are marked with a series of themes or codes, which are extracted from the text. The codes or themes are grouped into similar *concepts* to make them more workable. From these concepts, *categories* are formed, which are the basis for the creation of a *theory*, or a reverse-engineered hypothesis. This contradicts the traditional model of research, where the researcher chooses a theoretical framework and only then applies this model to the phenomenon to be studied (Glaser and Strauss 1967).

For example, one of our doctorate students, Isaac Narh, conducted a study in 2018 entitled 'Grounded theory exploration of the student nurse clinical learning environment supervision in the Greater Accra of Ghana'. As the student was unable to find any research papers on this topic in Ghana in the literature, he decided that the best design would be to use grounded theory so that he could come up with a theory about how the student nurses' clinical learning environment supervision was undertaken in Ghana.

Relating a specific research question to an appropriate research design

Having discussed the main types of quantitative and qualitative research designs, how does the specific type of research question relate to the appropriate research design? A summary of the types of research designs best suited to the different types of review questions can be found in Table 2.8.

Table 2.8 Summary of the types of research designs best suited to the different types of review questions

Type of question	Suggested type of study			
	Least biased ————————————————— Most biased			
Treatment or therapy	RCT >	cohort >	case-control >	case series
Diagnosis	Retrospective, blind comparison with gold standard			
Aetiology or harm	RCT >	cohort >	case-control >	case series
Prognosis		cohort >	case-control >	case series
Prevention	RCT >	cohort >	case-control >	case series
Experiences or perceptions	Qualitative studies: most common are phenomenological, ethnographic and grounded theory			

Questions of therapy, causes and prevention that can best be answered by RCTs can also be answered by meta-analysis and systematic reviews.

Qualitative questions where a significant amount of research on the same research question has been conducted can also be answered by systematic reviews.

Box 2.8   Levels of evidence

Level 1: Systematic reviews and meta-analysis of RCTs; evidence-based clinical practice guidelines

Level 2: One or more RCTs

Level 3: Controlled trials (no randomization)

Level 4: Case-control or cohort study

Level 5: Systematic review of descriptive and qualitative studies

Level 6: Single descriptive or qualitative study

Level 7: Expert opinion

A well-planned research design helps ensure that your methods match your research aims, that you collect high-quality data and that you use the right kind of analysis to answer your questions, utilizing credible sources. This allows you to draw valid, trustworthy conclusions. At this stage it is important to highlight that not all research designs are robust. It is widely accepted that some designs have more bias (the quality and rigour of the research systems and process followed) than others. This is depicted in the various levels and hierarchy of evidence, detailed in Box 2.8 and Figure 2.12.

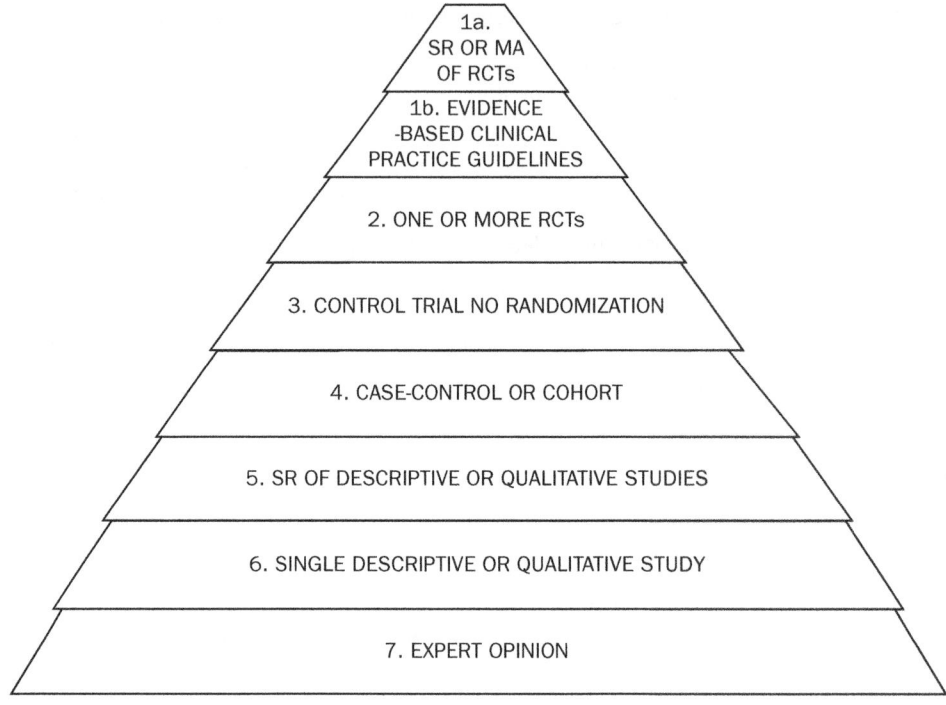

SR = Systematic Review; MA = Meta-analysis

Figure 2.12 Evidence pyramid.

🔑 Key points

- Selecting a topic area for your systematic review is the first step towards undertaking the review.
- The specific topic you select may arise from a number of different triggers.
- Once you have selected your review topic, the next step is to narrow this down to a specific review question.
- There are two main types of questions: background questions (general nursing questions) and foreground questions (answering a specific question about a specific topic).
- Foreground questions and sources can be divided into primary sources, such as original research, and secondary sources, such as systematic reviews.
- Formulating a review question is the most critical and perhaps the most difficult part of any systematic review.
- The review question underpins all the components of the review methods.
- It is important to ensure that you ask an open question. It is best to avoid closed questions that can be answered with a simple yes or no.
- The main types of review questions relate to treatment or therapy, prevention, diagnosis, prognosis, causation and experiences.

- It is important that your review question is both comprehensive and specific.
- A well-framed review question will have four or five elements. The review question formation usually includes identifying all the component parts: the population, the intervention or exposure, the comparative intervention (if any), the outcomes that are measured and the type of research design. The acronyms for these are PICOT or PEOT.
- It is important to match your review question to the appropriate research design.
- The research design can be thought of as the structure of the review question.
- There are different levels and hierarchy of evidence.

Summary

This chapter has discussed the different ways of finding topic areas for your systematic review and described the meaning and functions of an answerable and focused review question. The chapter presented the main types of focused review questions, together with some examples from nursing practice. The chapter discussed the different types of review questions and the importance of choosing the appropriate research design for the type of review question you have selected. A number of templates were provided to help you formulate your own answerable and focused systematic review question.

Questions and Answers (Q&A)

(Q) What can help you identify an area to focus a review question?

(A) An effective way of identifying an area to focus your review question is to look at what is topical in the nursing press and wider health and care sectors. Similarly, looking at the news headlines in specific journals may help you generate and focus your ideas. Finally, talking to colleagues in practice is a great way of identifying areas to focus on a review question.

(Q) Why is it important to develop the correct review question?

(A) Investing the time and effort to develop a sound review question will result in a better quality systematic review. For example, ensuring you have the best designs or plans for building a new house will ensure the foundations and building are strong and long-lasting. Similarly, by having a well-focused review question, your results and findings will be much more reliable.

References

Anastasiadis, E., Prabhakar, P. and Winchester, C.L. (2015) Framing a research question: The first and most vital step in planning research. *Journal of Clinical Urology* 8 (6): 409–411.

Bailey, D.M. (1997) *Research for the Health Professional: A Practical Guide*, 2nd edn. Philadelphia: F.A. Davis.

Blaikie, N. (2007) *Approaches to Social Enquiry*, 2nd edn. Cambridge: Polity Press.

Glaser, B.G. and Strauss, A. (1967) *Discovery of Grounded Theory: Strategies for Qualitative Research*. Mill Valley, CA: Sociology Press.

Greene, M. (1997) The lived world, literature and education. In D. Vandenberg (ed.) *Phenomenology and Educational Discourse*. Johannesburg: Heinemann.

Hissong, A., Lape, J.E. and Bailey, D.M. (2015) *Bailey's Research for the Health Professional*, 3rd ed. Philadelphia: F.A. Davis.

Hulley, B.S., Cummings, S., Browner, W., Grady, D. and Newman, T.B. (2007) Conceiving the research question. In *Designing Clinical Research*, 3rd edn. Philadelphia: Lippincott Williams & Wilkins.

Khan, K.S. and Zamora, J. (2022) *Systematic Reviews to Support Evidence-Based Medicine: How to Appraise, Conduct and Publish Reviews*, 3rd edn. Boca Raton, FL: CRC Press.

Noble, H. and Mitchell, G. (2016) What is grounded theory? *Evidence-Based Nursing* 19 (2): 34–35.

Pink, S., Horst, H., Postill, J., Hjorth, L., Lewis, T. and Tacchi, J. (2015) *Digital Ethnography: Principles and Practice*. London: Sage.

Schulz, K.F. and Grimes, D.A. (2002) Case-control studies: Research in reverse. *The Lancet* 359 (9304): 431–434.

Spradley, J.P. (1979) *The Ethnographic Interview*. New York: Holt, Rinehart and Winston.

Stanford University (n.d.) Advancing ethnographic and fieldwork research. Available at https://ethnographylab.stanford.edu/ (accessed 9 August 2023).

3

Creating the protocol for your systematic review

Overview

- The importance of writing a protocol for your review
- Steps to take when planning your review protocol
- Sections to include within your protocol
- Brief overview of all the steps/sections to include within your protocol

The importance of writing a protocol for your review

Writing a protocol of what you intend to include before you start your systematic review is very important. A protocol (also called a 'plan') describes in advance the review question and your rationale for the methods you will use. It also includes details of how different types of studies will be located, appraised and synthesized (Purssell and McCrae 2020). Describing your methods in advance is a way of trying to minimize bias (something that causes a consistent deviation from the truth), as you cannot start changing the way you review the papers once you see the results of the identified studies. For instance, if you said in the protocol that you will be including only RCTs and then found a study by a well-known nurse or healthcare professional which was not an RCT, the temptation might be for you to include it. However, you would not be able to do this, as you have stated otherwise in your protocol. Another important reason to undertake a protocol for your review is that you can then show this to colleagues, patients with the specific problem and/or your supervisor. They can read your protocol and provide you with further suggestions to improve it, as you may not have thought of relevant issues that are important to the patients, service users and other nurses and healthcare professionals (Khan and Zamora 2022).

Although most nurses who are conducting their first review will conduct it on their own, the highest quality systematic reviews, such as those undertaken by the Cochrane Centre, Campbell Collaboration and the Joanna Briggs Institute, are usually undertaken in teams. Conducting a review in a team decreases bias and increases the validity (or truthfulness) of the results. If you are a student nurse or a clinician without access to a team, it is perfectly acceptable for the purposes of academic study to conduct a review on your own, so long as you acknowledge that doing so may decrease the validity of your results and increase the level of bias in your review.

Practical Tip

If you are undertaking a systematic review on your own before preparing the protocol, always talk to professional colleagues and academic supervisors in your area about your proposed idea and reasons for the systematic review. This approach will help you formulate your ideas and enrich the protocol, which is essentially the blueprint for the systematic review.

Steps to take when planning your review protocol

Additionally, you may find it difficult to publish the work. Where possible we would recommend that you try to create your own review team by involving other students or members of your clinical team. This is important to enhance the screening and selection processes of your papers in preparing the final review.

Once you have formulated your review question, it is a good idea to undertake a quick general search (also called a scoping search) to make sure that there are no systematic literature reviews already available or in progress that have addressed your review question. Box 1.2 in Chapter 1 shows some common websites where you can check this out (please note that this list is not exhaustive). An excellent check-list can be found in a book called *Systematic Reviews* available from the Centre for Reviews and Dissemination (CRD) website (see Box 1.2).

Here are some useful tips and techniques to consider when searching the different websites:

- If you find a *narrative review* published on your topic and review question, first of all check the publication date. If the review was published five years ago or more, we would suggest that it would be acceptable to go ahead with your own systematic literature review. This is because the quality of systematic review is considered to be superior to a narrative review.

- If you find a systematic literature review or reviews that are exactly like the one your protocol aims to carry out, there are a number of strategies you can follow:

  o You could look to see if the review or reviews you found were conducted recently or a number of years previously. If a number of primary papers on the specific review question have been published since the last systematic review, it is still fine to go ahead with your own systematic review. This is based on the premise that your review will update any previous review by furthering new knowledge.

  o If no new reviews have been published since the last systematic review, there is no point in conducting a review that would produce exactly the same results. The best thing to do in this case is to *change* or *tweak* the **P**opulation group, the **I**ntervention, the **C**omparative group, the **O**utcomes or **T**ype of research design, so your specific review question will be different to the previously published systematic review. For example, in the case study of Tamara (in Box 2.3 in Chapter 2), her title is: 'In patients with adolescent idiopathic scoliosis, how effective is spinal bracing and scoliosis-specific exercises compared with other treatments at reducing spinal curvature, rib hump and psychological problems?' If she found a systematic literature review that had already been conducted and no new primary papers had been published since, she could change the population group and look at adults. Alternatively, she could look at a subgroup of the population, such as obese adolescents, or change the intervention, comparative group or specific outcomes to be investigated.

Practice session 3.1

For your own review question, search the websites provided in Box 1.2 in Chapter 1 to identify whether your review question has already been addressed through a systematic review.

Sections to include within your protocol

The length of time you devote to writing up your protocol depends on the specific circumstances under which you are writing your review. If you are writing up the review to answer a review question for yourself, it is acceptable for the protocol of your review to be quite brief and sketchy, but it still needs to contain all the essentials detailed below. If you are proposing a protocol for a more formal review – for instance if you are conducting this review as part of your continuing professional development or if it is a requirement for a module on a formal undergraduate or postgraduate nursing programme, such as a dissertation – the protocol of your review will need to be comprehensively detailed, logically sequenced and precise.

Practical Tip

Investing the time and effort to devise a sound protocol at this early stage will only serve to enhance the quality and outcomes, along with increasing the chances of publishing your systematic review.

Brief overview of all the steps/sections to include within your protocol

A summary of what should be included in each step of your review protocol is found below. The sections within the protocol and the full review are similar, except that in the protocol, they do not include the results and discussion sections that are presented in the final systematic review (University of Reading n.d.). An overview of all the sections to include within your protocol (and later your full systematic review) is listed below. Chapters 4–12 in this book provide a much more detailed discussion of the full process for conducting each section of the systematic review. Full details for undertaking each part of the review can be found in the chapters indicated below.

Step 1: Developing an answerable review question (Chapter 2)

This has been discussed in Chapter 2.

 ### Step 2: Writing your protocol (Chapter 3)

This step is detailed in this chapter.

 ### Step 3: Writing the background to your systematic review (Chapter 4)

The background section of a systematic review is similar to writing a narrative review. The purpose of the background section is to provide an overview of the specific area of the review, highlighting the clinical problems associated with the area or question, and to discuss the relevant reviews within the specific clinical area in order to identify the gap in systematic reviews in this area.

 ### Step 4: Writing the objectives (or purpose of the systematic review) (Chapter 5)

The purpose of writing the objectives of your review is to clarify your reason for conducting the systematic review.

 ### Step 5: Specifying your inclusion and exclusion criteria (Chapter 5)

In this section you need to decide on the specific criteria by which your protocol aims to select (or not select) the primary papers for your systematic review. These will include specific criteria on the types of subjects, interventions (or exposure), comparative group and outcomes, as well as the types of studies to include and exclude in the protocol and subsequent systematic review.

 ### Step 6: Conducting the search strategy (Chapter 6)

The search strategy describes how and where your protocol relates to searching for primary research papers to include in your systematic review. To ensure that your search strategy is replicable, it is important to include a detailed description of your search strategy that is based on the PICOT (population, intervention, comparative group or intervention, outcome and type of study) or PEOT (patient, exposure, outcome and type of study) of your review question (see Chapter 2 for more on these acronyms).

 ### Step 7: Selecting (Chapter 7) appraising (Chapter 8) and extracting (Chapter 9) the relevant data from your primary research papers to answer your review question

In this section you need to describe how your protocol will aid you in selecting and evaluating papers, along with identifying the framework you plan to use. The process of extracting data from your papers to answer the review question also needs to be articulated. In other words, you will be explaining in detail how your protocol will help you to go through the chosen papers and take out the relevant information to answer your review question. Full details of how to do this are outlined in Chapters 7–9.

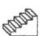 ### Step 8: Plans for synthesizing, summarizing and presenting the data (Chapter 10)

In this step of the protocol, it is important to describe the methods that you plan to use to synthesize your data (both the qualitative as well as the quantitative data if you are conducting a mixed-methods systematic review).

 ### Step 9: Writing up your discussion and completing your review (Chapter 11)

With the exceptions of steps 7, 8 and 9, all the remaining chapters need to be included in the protocol. At this point the protocol is written in the future tense. However, on completing the full review you will need to detail the processes undertaken (in the past tense).

Fay: An example of a student's systematic review protocol

The rest of this chapter provides an example of a real student's systematic review dissertation, following feedback from readers, so that you can see for yourself what a protocol may look like. Please note that as the content of the example protocol may now be dated and the rules and regulations mentioned within this example may now have changed, we would like you to concentrate mainly on the format and not so much on the content. We have included authors' names within the body of the protocol for illustration purposes only. We have not therefore included the full references for the protocol in the book. If you are considering a similar review we would recommend you start at the beginning. Please note that the student gave their permission for their work to be used as an example.

Fay was studying for a Bachelor of Science (BSc) in Nursing several years ago. This example protocol is only intended to *illustrate* how a protocol can be developed and may therefore not be reflective of current policy and practice, evidence, and standards and competences. The area of interest of the student conducting this systematic review was urinary tract infections (UTIs) and the aim of the systematic review was to evaluate the existing guidelines that promote the practice of *not* using antiseptics at catheter insertion. The review question was: 'In patients requiring urinary catherization, is sterile catheter insertion more effective than non-sterile insertion at reducing the incidence of catheter-associated urinary tract infection (CAUTI)?' The text that follows has been taken from her review protocol.

Step 1: Developing an answerable review question/title (Chapter 2)

Example: Fay's protocol, front cover

Review question: In patients requiring urinary catheterization, is sterile catheter insertion more effective than non-sterile insertion at reducing the incidence of catheter-associated urinary tract infection (CAUTI)?

Commentary on writing the review title or question

As you may observe above, the review title is written as a review question. Ideally it needs to be a statement.

Step 1: The review question should be broken down into the component parts as specified by the PICOT or PEOT framework: in patients requiring urinary catheterization **(P)**, is sterile catheter insertion **(I)** more effective than non-sterile insertion **(C)** at reducing the incidence of catheter-associated urinary tract infections (CAUTIs) **(O)**? To change it to a statement you could write it as follows: A comparison of sterile **(I)** versus non-sterile catheterization **(C)** in patients requiring catheterization **(P)** to reduce the incidence of infections in patients **(O)** with catheter-associated urinary tract infections: A comparative study **(T)**

Additionally, an important point to consider is that when writing a high-quality Cochrane or Campbell review, it is recommended that you write the background for an intervention review under four main headings:

Description of the condition

Description of the intervention

How the intervention might work

Why it is important to do this review

 Step 2 is the completed protocol

 Step 3: Background and description of the condition

Urinary catheterization of patients is a common nursing procedure used both in the hospital and in the community. According to Dougherty and Lister (2004, pg 333) catheter-associated infections are the most common nosocomial infection, counting up to around 45% of all hospital-acquired infections. Hospital-acquired infection can be defined as an infection that is neither present, nor incubating, at the time of admission to hospital (Hospital Acquired Infection [online]). Studies by Bryan and Reynolds (1984, pg 494–498) and Turck and Stamm (1981, pg 651–654) concluded that between 75% and 80% of all healthcare-associated UTIs follow the insertion of a urinary catheter and a study by Glynn et al (1997), which investigated 40 English hospitals, estimated that around 26% of all hospitalized patients have a urinary catheter inserted, whilst Parker (1999, pg 563–574) and Godfrey and Evans (2000, pg 682–690) suggest that 4% of patients in the community, at some point, will have a catheter inserted. Furthermore, complications that may arise from urinary catheterization include structural damage to the urinary tract, bleeding, false passage, and urinary tract infections and bacteriuria (Joanna Briggs). It is estimated that CAUTI costs the National Health Service (NHS) £1,327 per patient and because it increases the period of hospitalization of such patients by approximately three to six days, costs approximately increase by £124 million per year (Hart, 2008, pg 44–48; SSHAIP, 2004, [online]).

Description of the intervention: Catheterization – types and indications

A catheter is a tubular device which is passed through the urethra into the bladder in order to drain urine or to instill medical treatment (Dougherty and Lister, 2004, pg 330–333; Steward, in BJN monograph, 2001, pg 42). Catheterization is indicated in and used to relieve obstructed flow of urine, to measure the residual amount in the bladder, to provide post-operative drainage following bladder, vaginal and prostate surgery, in monitoring hourly urine output in the critically ill patient, and in continence care (Brunner and Suddarth, 1992, pg 682; Steward, in BJN monograph, 2001, pg 42). Insertion of a urinary catheter is a common procedure in both acute and primary care settings, and careful consideration is always required over the need for, versus, the risk of this procedure. Urethral catheterization may be performed as an indwelling or an intermittent procedure. Indwelling catheterization consists of continuous catheter drainage which can be sub-classified into short term (1–7 days), mid-term (7–28 days) and long term (28 days up to 3 months) (Hart, 2008, pg 44–48; Head, 2006, pg 33–36;RCN, 2008, pg 2–55). Intermittent catheterization consists of episodic introduction of a catheter into the bladder to drain urine out (Dougherty and Lister, 2004, pg 335). The catheter is passed via the urethra and removed soon after the bladder urine is drained. In recent years this technique has become noticeably popular, and can be carried out by the patient him/herself or by the nurse. This form of catheterization is indicated for the drainage of a poorly functioning bladder (as is found in spinal cord injury patients and those with neurological disorders) and for urinary drainage in the peri-operative period. Its main advantage is that the patient is left catheter-free in between catheterizations (Dougherty and Lister, 2004, pg 335; Robinson, 2007, pg 48–56). Intermittent catheterization is also commonly used to instill medications, measure residual urine, and it is also used to instill contrast material into the bladder to study the bladder and the urethra (Hart, 2008, pg 44–48). Lapides et al. (2002, pg 1584–1586) and Wilson (1998, pg S10–13) advocate that this procedure should be undertaken as a sterile procedure in the hospital environment due to the high risk of hospital-acquired infections, while in the community a clean technique should be used.

Catheter-associated urinary tract infection

Catheters are a major cause of urinary tract infection; they pave the way for microorganisms to enter the bladder. Since they are a foreign body they consequently offer a surface for micro-organisms to grow on and act as a route for microorganisms to gain access into the urinary tract. Insertion may result in physical damage to the urethra and catheters may interfere with the body's immune responses and may cause a chemical-induced inflammation in the urethral and bladder mucosa (Walsh, 1997, pg 672). All these factors are responsible for predisposing to CAUTI. Catheter-associated urinary tract infections may affect any part of the urinary system and are caused by exogenous microorganisms or endogenous faecal or urethral microorganisms (Godfrey and Evans, 2000, pg 682–690). Saint and Lipsky (1999, pg 800–808) suggest that these infections can also be acquired by cross-contamination from other patients or hospital healthcare workers or by exposure to contaminated solutions or non-sterile equipment. The normal urinary tract is least sterile near the urethral orifice; hence, microorganisms can inhabit the meatus or distal urethra and thus be introduced directly into the bladder on catheter insertion (Parker, 1999, pg 563–574). In long-term indwelling catheterization microorganisms may enter the urinary tract through two possible routes, from the catheter lumen (intraluminal infection) or via the space between the walls of the catheter and the urethra (the periurethral or extraluminal route) (Getliffe, 1996, pg 548–554). Therefore shorter periods of catheterization and minimal catheter and drainage bag handling are recognized forms of preventing such infections (Mangnall and Waterson, 2006, pg 49–56). Alexander et al. (2000, pg 319) indicate that urinary infections are most common in females. The female urethra is shorter and its external meatus is closer to the perineal area and thus offers a shorter distance for microbes to reach the urinary tract (Tambyah, 2004, pg S44–S48).

CAUTI is asymptomatic in the majority of cases (Tambyah et al, 2000, pg 678–682); however, Godfrey and Evans (2000, pg 682–690) clarify that CAUTI can present with signs and symptoms such as pyrexia, pyuria, urinary bypassing of the catheter, cloudy foul-smelling urine, confusion in elderly patients, haematuria and back pain. These symptoms may vary with the age and sex of the patient and also with the severity and site of the infection. Pickerman (1994, pg 66–68) suggests that these signs and symptoms occur when the bacteria invade the bladder mucosa resulting in inflammation. Diagnosis is established after obtaining a urine sample for culture and sensitivity. A bacterial count of 100,000 organisms (or CFU) per millilitre is considered to be significant of urinary tract infection. Bacteriuria and urinary tract infection are two terms used interchangeably in the nursing literature. Bacteriuria is the presence of bacteria in the urine; however, according to Higgins (1995, pg 33–35) bacteriuria in patients with indwelling and intermittent catheters does not always suggest a diagnosis of urinary tract infection (UTI).

How the intervention might work: Guidelines on catheterization technique

Guidelines by both the Royal College of Nurses (RCN, 2008, pg 42–45) and the National Institute for Health and Clinical Excellence (NIHCE, 2003, pg 8–11) emphasize the use of aseptic technique at catheter insertion in order to prevent catheter-associated urinary tract infection. This recommended aseptic technique is mainly a non-touch procedure which involves preparation of the environment and equipment, and hand washing, which is considered to be most effective at reducing the risk of hospital-acquired infection (DoH, 2001, pg S21–37; Gould et al, 2007, pg 109–115). It also involves the use of sterile gloves and disposable aprons; Callaghan (1998, pg 37–420) points out that disposable aprons are worn to protect nurses' clothing from contamination, and thus reduce the risk of transferring microorganisms to other patients. The NMC (2008) suggests cleaning of the meatal area with sterile agents and use of sterile lubricating gel in order to make catheterization more comfortable and reduce the risk of urethral trauma. However, Dougherty and Lister (2004, pg 333–334) consider vigorous meatal cleaning as unnecessary; on the other hand, Tambyah et al. (1999, pg 131–136) emphasize that infection occurs extraluminally on catheter insertion, and thus suggest that antiseptic cleaning of the meatus is vital. Leaver (2007, pg 39–42) also states that meatal cleansing mechanically removes exudates and smegma.

Why is it important to do this review? Rationale of the study

Opinions as to the choice of meatal cleansing solution (whether it is an antiseptic or a simple sterile solution) and how sterile the whole procedure of catheter insertion should be have varied over time and from region to region. Other national guidelines found in documents such as Winning Ways (DH 2003) and Essential Steps to Safe, Clean Care (DH 2006) are aimed at reducing risks of and the incidence of healthcare-associated infections (HCAI). These documents are based on the NIHCE guidelines (2003) which in turn have been based on EPIC guidelines developed by Pratt et al. (2001). The latter guidelines were updated in EPIC 2, which was published in 2006. Although such publications strive to present clear information on what needs to be done in specific situations to reduce risks, it seems that they may remain open to interpretation if they are not based on solid reliable evidence. EPIC's (Pratt et al., 2006, pg S30) recommendations on cleaning the urethral meatus using sterile normal saline and using sterile non-antiseptic lubricating gel were, as admitted by the authors, based on expert opinion. It is no wonder, therefore, that the type of cleansing solution to be used is not even mentioned in the RCN guidelines (RCN, 2008), and the NIHCE guidelines (2003) leave the choice of cleansing solution to the healthcarer and recommend adherence to local guidelines and policies. Pellowe (2004, pg 13–14) suggests that detailed operational protocols at local level must incorporate such guidelines and principles for preventing HCAIs such as CAUTI. Furthermore, as evidenced by comments in a letter to the editor (Panknin and Althaus, 2001, pg 146–147) that criticizes EPIC's decision on including their recommendation on meatal cleansing when it was based only on expert opinion, the opinion in other countries in Europe regarding disinfection of the meatal area disagrees with guidelines in this country. The authors of this letter claim that antiseptic disinfection is the norm in their institution and in their opinion it explains their lower incidence of CAUTI.

Three systematic reviews were identified in the literature. The review by Jamison et al. (2004) focuses mainly on the use of catheter types in management of the neurogenic bladder, whereas the review by Niel-Weise and Van den Broek (2005) looked at studies comparing urethral indwelling, intermittent and supra-pubic catheterization. The review by Lockwood et al. (2004, pg 271–291) treated the issue of sterility at insertion very briefly; only two relevant studies were included. Since these reviews focused mainly on other catheter-related matters, their search strategy could have resulted in studies relevant to the antiseptic issue being missed and left out. This study focused solely on this particular issue of sterility at catheter insertion and adopted a search strategy that would include as many of the studies that specifically dealt with this topic.

Step 3: Aims and objectives

The aim of this review was to establish whether urinary catheterization performed using a strict sterile technique is more effective than a non-sterile insertion technique at reducing the incidence of CAUTI in patients requiring urinary catheterization. Evidence from studies dealing with sterile/non-sterile insertion techniques and more specifically the steps involved in it (i.e. antiseptic periurethral cleaning, hand washing and sterile gloves, with sterile or antiseptic-containing lubricating gel) have been evaluated. The objective of this study, hence, is to identify the relevant literature that exists that could serve as evidence that would settle this discrepancy in opinion.

Step 4: Criteria for considering studies for this review

The criteria for the selection of studies to be included in a review need to be defined ahead of the selection process in order to avoid selection bias (Khan et al. 2003, pg 29). The components of the structured question are used to generate a list of selection criteria. Using the PICO (Population, Intervention, Comparison and Outcome) framework facilitates the process. The study types or designs are identified after considering their likely suitability for answering the review question and their level on the evidence hierarchy, while also bearing in mind the probable abundance or sparsity of the relevant studies. Torgerson (2003, pg 27–28) recommends a rapid scope of the literature early in the planning stage to establish how plentiful relevant studies are. This also serves to identify existing reviews; however, Torgerson also warns that this could be a source of bias in the review.

Types of studies

The best study designs to answer review questions regarding effectiveness of an intervention are comparative studies; these studies compare the effect of the intervention on outcomes in the study group with outcomes in the control group (who are not exposed to the intervention being assessed). Randomized controlled trials (RCTs) feature high on the hierarchy of evidence when allocation to the two groups is randomized and concealed; bias is avoided since any confounding variables are equally distributed between the two groups (Craig and Smyth 2002, pg 89–92). However, following a rapid scope of the literature, it was evident that studies relevant to the review question were unlikely to be numerous; therefore it was deemed necessary to include other designs (shown in Table 3.1) that are not considered as sound as RCTs.

The participants

Patients who required and underwent urinary catheterization, whether indwelling (short term or long term) or intermittent, and which was performed by a healthcarer were included in the review. However, patients who underwent intermittent self-catheterization were excluded, along with those having pre-existing urinary tract infections, those who had undergone urological surgery and those who were on antibiotics.

Types of intervention

The interventions under investigation were the sterile or aseptic catheter insertion technique and the specific steps involved in the process, namely hand washing, sterile gloves and gowns, antiseptic meatal cleansing and use of antiseptic lubricating gel.

Types of comparison

Non-sterile or clean catheter insertion techniques were the comparisons or controls examined; these included insertion techniques or their component steps that did not use antiseptics or sterile equipment as is used in the sterile technique. Also included were insertion techniques where one or more of the specific steps of the sterile approach were either omitted or modified and/or where any of the following occurred:

- Hand washing is omitted or modified and/or
- no sterile gloves are used and/or
- no sterile gowns are used and/or
- no antiseptic meatal cleansing and/or
- the lubricating gel used contains no antiseptic.

Types of outcome measures

The rate of incidence of CAUTI was considered as the outcome measure. CAUTI was identified as established by the presence of its clinical symptoms and/or the presence of significant bacteriuria. Significant bacteriuria was defined as 100,000 CFU/ml and was considered to be more reliable at diagnosing CAUTI, since the latter may be asymptomatic. It was assumed that CAUTI that could, safely, be attributed directly to catheter insertion would occur within the first few days following insertion and hence urine samples showing significant bacteriuria within this period would be most reliable.

Inclusion/exclusion criteria

A summary of the inclusion/exclusion criteria can be seen in Table 3.1.

F **Table 3.1** Inclusion and exclusion criteria

	Inclusion criteria	Exclusion criteria
Population	Male or female patients undergoing urinary catheterization performed by healthcarers Short-term/long-term indwelling or intermittent catheterization Setting: hospital, rehabilitation unit or nursing home	Intermittent self-catheterization, suprapubic catheterization, pre-existing urinary tract infection, urological surgery, patients on anitbiotics
Intervention	Sterile urethral catheterization	Other forms of catheterization
Comparison	Non-sterile urethral catheterization	Other forms of catheterization
Outcome	CAUTI confirmed by significant bacteriuria or clinical symptoms or urethral colony counts	Any other outcomes
Study design	Comparative studies: randomized controlled studies, non-randomized experimental studies and observational studies with control group	Studies without control groups

Step 5: The search strategy

Introduction

The search strategy ensures that the literature searching is as wide and thorough as is possible; thus all or most of the relevant evidence that exists and that can address the research question is identified and analysed. A comprehensive search by reducing both uncertainty and bias ensures precision and validity of the review (Khan et al. 2003, pg 21–22). This step identifies the literature sources that were searched and the process of generating a search term combination for electronic database searches.

The literature sources

Both electronic and manual searches will be performed to find all the relevant studies. The grey literature, which according to Polit and Beck (2006, pg 480) consists of unpublished reports, dissertations, non-referenced publications and any other studies with similar limited distribution, were also searched for along with any ongoing research.

The electronic searches

The electronic databases shown in Table 3.2 will be searched using the search strategy list shown in Figure 3.1; a full explanation of the way this list was generated is in the next section of this chapter. All searches will be saved online for future reference and printed copies will be included. The hits obtained and the potentially relevant studies and their abstracts that will be found will be recorded and documented.

F **Table 3.2** List of electronic databases

Database	Description	Dates covered
(OVID Host) Journals @ Ovid Full text	OVIDONLINE	Up to 2 Sept 2008
Ovid MEDLINE (R)		1950 to August 2008
Ovid MEDLINE (R)	In-process & other non-indexed citations and Ovid MEDLINE (R)	1950 to present
CINAHL	CINAHL – Cumulative Index to Nursing & Allied Health Literature	1982 to August 2008
AMED	Allied and Complementary Medicine	1985 to August 2008
EMBASE		1988 to Week 35 2008
EBM Reviews	All EBM Reviews – Cochrane DSR, ACP Journal Club, DARE, CCTR, CMR, HTA and NHSEED	1991 to August 2008
BNI	British Nursing Index and Archive	1985 to August 2008

Hand searches

Manual searches will be performed by:

- scanning the reference lists of all related studies
- searching for grey literature by searching the internet, in particular the following gateways and search engines: http://www.webarchive.org.uk/wayback/archive/20140614081921/http://www.jisc.ac.uk/whatwedo/programmes/reppres/irs.aspx (Intute Repository Search [IRS] project); https://www.shef.ac.uk/scharr (School of Health and Related Research); http://www.google.com/scholar
- searching the following search engines/databases for conference proceedings and papers, dissertations and theses, and expertise: https://portal.nihr.ac.uk; http://www.cos.com/; http://www.bl.uk
- searching for any possible ongoing research on the following databases: www.york.ac.uk/inst/crd/htadbase.htm; http://controlled-trials.com.

The search term strategy list

The list of search terms and combinations shown in Figure 3.1 will be used to search the electronic databases. It is based on the research question and its PICO components. The sensitivity of the search, which according to Khan et al. (2003, pg 24) is the proportion of relevant studies, is higher when synonyms to the component terms are included in the list. It is also increased by including abbreviations and spelling variants of the terms. Khan et al. (2003, pg 24) emphasize that sensitivity is a reflection of the comprehensiveness of the search. On the other hand the precision of the search, defined by Khan et al. (2003, pg 27) as the number of relevant studies identified expressed as a percentage of all studies identified (relevant and not), is increased by combinations of the terms using Boolean operators and by applying limits. In order to make the search more specific, at the end of the literature search the following limits were applied: English language, human, humans and research.

Generation of the search term and combination list

The generation of the search terms and combination of lists will involve seven stages to arrive at the final search strategy list.

> **Stage 1: Review question.** The structured question will be broken down into the component parts as specified by the PICO framework: in *Patients requiring urinary catheterization* **(P)**, is *sterile catheter insertion* **(I)** more effective than *non-sterile insertion* **(C)** at reducing the incidence of *catheter-associated urinary tract infections (CAUTIs)* **(O)**?

> **Stage 2: Keywords and phrases.** Using the PICO groups, keywords and phrases were identified, which are displayed in Table 3.3.

> **Stage 3: Identification of synonyms.** The synonyms of the search terms that were identified can be seen in Table 3.4.

F **Table 3.3** Keywords and phrases

Population	Intervention	Comparison	Outcome	Types of study designs
Patients requiring urinary catheterization	Sterile catheter insertion	Non-sterile catheter	Catheter-associated infection	Comparative studies: randomized controlled studies, non-randomized experimental studies and observational studies with control group

F **Table 3.4** Synonyms of keywords and phrases

Population	Intervention	Comparison	Outcome
Urinary catheterization	Sterile	Non-sterile	Urinary tract infection
Urethral catheterization	Aseptic	Clean	Bladder infection
Bladder catheterization	Periurethral cleansing	Water	Infection
Catheterization	Meatal cleansing	Saline	Bacteriuria
Catheter insertion	Chlorhexidine	Gloves	Asymptomatic bacteriuria
	Cetrimide		Significant bacteriuria
	Savlon		Urine dipslide
	Povidone-iodine		Dipslide
	Antiseptic solution		Urine culture
	Antiseptic		Urine sample
	Gloves		
	Gel		
	Lubricating gel		
	Antiseptic gel		
	Hand washing		
	Hand hygiene		

Stage 4: Combining keywords and phrases. At this step the type of study design/s was included and using Boolean operators (OR, AND, NOT) the combinations of terms will be obtained; these are presented in Table 3.5.

F **Table 3.5** Combinations of keywords and phrases

Population Boolean Operators	Intervention AND	Comparison AND	Outcome AND	Study designs AND
OR Urinary catheterisation	Sterile	Non-sterile	Urinary tract infection	Comparative
OR Urethral catheterisation	Aseptic	Clean	Bladder infection	Randomised
OR Bladder catheterisation	Periurethral cleansing	Water	Infection	Controlled
OR Catheterisation	Meatal cleansing	Saline	Bacteriuria	Quasi-randomised
OR Catheter insertion	Chlorhexidine	Gloves	Asymptomatic bacteriuria	Observational
OR	Cetrimide		Significant bacteriuria	Study
OR	Savlon		Urine dipslide	Trial
OR	Povidone-iodine		Dipslide	Quantitative
OR	Antiseptic solution		Urine culture	RCT
OR	Antiseptic		Urine sample	
OR	Gloves			
OR	Gel			
OR	Lubricating gel			
OR	Antiseptic gel			
OR	Hand washing			
OR	Hand hygiene			

Stage 5: Identifying abbreviations and different spellings. Possible abbreviations or spelling variants (Americanisms) of the terms in Stage 4 will be considered and the changes, displayed in Table 3.6, were obtained using truncation ($) and wild cards (?); these changes increase the sensitivity of the search.

Stage 6: Constructing a search strategy table. In Table 3.7 all of the terms were numbered, starting with the first term in the first column on the left.

F **Table 3.6** Abbreviations and different spellings

Population Boolean operators	Intervention AND	Comparison AND	Outcome AND	Study designs AND
OR Urinary catheteri?ation	Sterile	Non-sterile	Urinary tract infection	Comparative
OR Urethral catheteri?ation	Aseptic	Clean	Bladder infection	Randomi?$
OR Bladder catheteri?ation	Periurethral clean?ing	Water	Infection$	Control?ed
OR Catheteri?$	Meatal clean?ing	Saline	Bacter?uria	Quasi-randomi?ed
OR Catheter insertion	Chlorhexidine	Glove$	Asymptomatic bacter?uria	Observational
OR	Cetrimide		Significant bacter?uria	Stud$
OR	Savlon		Urine dipslide	Trial$
OR	Povidoneiodine		Dipslide	Quantitative
OR	Antiseptic solution$		Urine culture$	RCT
OR	Antiseptic$		Urine sample$	
OR	Glove$		CAUTI	
OR	Gel		UTI	
OR	Lubricating gel			
OR	Antiseptic gel			
OR	Hand washing			
OR	Hand hygiene			

A number was skipped on progressing from one column to the next; these numbers were then allocated to the combinations, as seen in Figure 3.1.

Stage 7: Translating into a search terms and combinations list. The resulting search term list can be seen in Figure 3.1. Where a search was carried out for a combination of terms, the Boolean search functions 'OR' and 'AND' are used (for example see item 6 in Figure 3.1, where OR has been used). The '?' is used as a wild card symbol. It replaces a single letter in a search word to find alternative spellings and plurals (for example orthop* will find both orthopaedic and orthopaedic), which is useful to detect American spellings.

F Table 3.7 Search strategy table

Population Boolean Operators	Intervention AND	Comparison AND	Outcome AND	Study designs AND
OR 1.Urinary catheteri?ation	7. Sterile	24. Non-sterile	30. Urinary tract infection	43. Comparative
OR 2. Urethral catheteri?ation	8. Aseptic	25. Clean	31. Bladder infection	44. Randomi?$
OR 3. Bladder catheteri?ation	9. Periurethral clean?ing	26. Water	32. Infection$	45. Control?ed
OR 4. Catheteri?$	10. Meatal clean?ing	27. Saline	33. Bacter?uria	46. Quasi-randomi?ed
OR 5. Catheter insertion	11. Chlorhexidine	28. Glove$	34. Asymptomatic bacter?uria	47.Observational
OR	12. Cetrimide		35. Significant bacter?uria	48. Stud$
OR	13. Savlon		36. Urine dipslide	49. Trial$
OR	14. Povidone-iodine		37. Dipslide	50. Quantitative
OR	15. Antiseptic solution$		38. Urine culture$	51. RCT
OR	16. Antiseptic$		39. Urine sample$	
OR	17. Glove$		40. CAUTI	
OR	18. Gel		41. UTI	
OR	19. Lubricating gel			
OR	20. Antiseptic gel			
OR	21. Hand washing			
OR	22. Hand hygiene			

The search term strategy list

---

1. Urinary catheteri?ation	23. 7 OR 8 OR 9 OR 10	39. Urine sample$
2. Urethral catheteri?ation	OR 11 OR 12 OR 13	40. CAUTI
3. Bladder catheteri?ation	OR 14 OR 15 OR 16	41. UTI
4. Catheteri?$	OR 17 OR 18 OR 19	42. 30 OR 31 OR 32
5. Catheter insertion	OR 20 OR 21 OR 22	OR 33 OR 34 OR 35
6. 1 OR 2 OR 3 OR 4 OR 5	24. Non-sterile	OR 36 OR 37
7. Sterile	25. Clean	OR 38 OR 39 OR 40
8. Aseptic	26. Water	OR 41
9. Periurethral clean?ing	27. Saline	43. Comparative
10. Meatal clean?ing	28. Glove$	44. Randomi?$
11. Chlorhexidine	29. 24 OR 25 OR 26 OR	45. Control?ed
12. Cetrimide	27 OR 28	46. Quasi-randomi?ed
13. Savlon	30. Urinary tract infection	47. Observational
14. Povidone-iodine	31. Bladder infection	48. Stud$
15. Antiseptic solution$	32. Infection$	49. Trial$
16. Antiseptic$	33. Bacter?uria	50. Quantitative
17. Glove$	34. Asymptomatic	51. RCT
18. Gel	bacter?uria	52. 43 OR 44 OR 45 OR
19. Lubricating gel	35. Significant bacter?uria	46 OR 47 OR 48 OR
20. Antiseptic gel	36. Urine dipslide	49 OR 50 OR 51
21. Hand washing	37. Dipslide	53. 6 AND 23 AND 29
22. Hand hygiene	38. Urine culture$	AND 42 AND 52

Figure 3.1 The search term strategy list.

The above list is identical to Table 3.7 but it also includes the combinations of the terms with AND and OR.

 Step 6: Selecting, appraising and extracting data from your primary research papers

Introduction

This section of the report will deal with the methods of the three phases of the review: the study selection process, the assessment of the methodological qualities of the selected studies and the data extraction process. All three phases of this review will be carried out solely by the author because of restrictions of time and work constraints. Ideally two reviewers working independently should be involved in order to reduce selection bias (Torgerson 2003, pg 40). Khan et al. (2003, pg 32) explain that the method of resolving any disagreements or undecided conclusions would need to be identified and would normally be clearly stated early in the protocol stage. Furthermore, agreement or consensus in most instances is reached through discussion; however, arbitration by a third person might be required if no agreed conclusion is reached.

Selection of studies

This consisted of two steps or stages. In the first step, the decision to include or exclude studies resulting from the search will be on the title and abstract only. In order to facilitate the process a standardized form will be used. This form was generated after considering the list of inclusion and exclusion criteria shown in Table 3.1 and therefore follows the PICO framework. Khan et al. (2003, pg 32) highlight the probability that decisions concerning inclusion/exclusion of studies can be highly subjective and therefore lead to disagreements when more than one reviewer is involved. Therefore, the use of standardized forms serves the secondary purpose of improving inter- and intra-rater reliability by ensuring that all reviewers' assessments follow a standardized systematic approach.

In the second step, a final decision on inclusion or exclusion of the studies identified in the first stage will be made, based on reading the full text; once again a standardized form will be used. The standardized forms used in the first and second selections had a similar basic layout, as shown in Tables 3.8 and 3.9. They consist of a list of questions that seek to identify those studies that meet the selection criteria. If all questions were answered in the affirmative, the study was included for assessment in the following

Table 3.8 Standardized form for first selection of studies (based on titles and abstracts)

Details of Study 1:

TITLE:

Authors:

Source:

Reviewer's name: Fay
Date:

	Criteria	Yes/no/undecided
Participants	Patients undergoing catheterization?	
	Type of catheterization: urethral, indwelling or intermittent?	
	Catheterization performed by healthcarer?	
	Setting: hospital or nursing home?	
Intervention	Sterile/aseptic catheter insertion, non-sterile/clean catheter insertion?	
Outcome	Incidence of CAUTI or bacteriuria	
Type of study	Quantitative, comparative?	
Action (with rationale)	Include (read full article) or exclude?	

F **Table 3.9** Standardized form for second selection of studies (based on full text)

Details of Study 1:

TITLE:

Authors:

Source:

Reviewer's name: Fay
Date:

	Criteria	Yes/no
Participants	Patients undergoing catheterization?	
	Type of catheterization: urethral, indwelling or intermittent?	
	Catheterization performed by healthcarer?	
	Setting: hospital or nursing home?	
Intervention	Sterile/aseptic catheter insertion, non-sterile/clean catheter insertion?	
Outcome	Incidence of CAUTI or bacteriuria	
Type of study	Quantitative, comparative?	
Action (with rationale)	Include (for full methodological analysis) or exclude?	

phase, but if all questions were answered in the negative such studies were obviously excluded. Any studies that ended up with an undecided conclusion in the first stage required further consideration by reading the full text before arriving at a final decision.

Assessment of methodological quality of included studies

The main objective of this assessment will be to establish the external and internal validity and reliability of the selected studies. According to Khan et al. (2003, pg 126) external validity, also known as generalizability, is the extent to which the effects observed in the study can be expected to apply in routine clinical practice, whereas internal validity refers to the degree to which the results of a study are likely to approximate the truth for the participants in the study (Khan et al., 2003, pg 132). The selected studies will be quantitative, comparative studies (that have a control group). The assessment tool or checklist that will be used to analyse these studies is based on the critical review form designed by Law et al. (1998) at McMaster University, originally intended for analysis of quantitative research studies related to occupational therapy. The adapted version of this form was chosen because it can be applied in analysis of all types of quantitative study designs and has a set of very detailed guidelines that makes it easier to use and increases its inter- and intra-rater reliability. The first page of a completed appraisal form for one of the included studies is shown in Figure 3.2.

Critical Review Form - Quantitative Studies
Law, M., Stewart, D., Pollock, N., Letts, L., Bosch, J., & Westmorland, M.

McMaster University

Adapted Word Version Used with Permission

The EB Group would like to thank Dr. Craig Scanlan, University of Medicine and Dentistry of NJ, for providing this Word version of the quantitative review form.

Instructions: Use tab or arrow keys to move between fields,mouse or spacebar to check/uncheck boxes.

CITATION	Provide the full citation for this article in APA format: Carapeti, E.A., Andrews, S.M. and Bentley, P.G. (1996) **Randomised study of sterile versus non-sterile urethral catheterisation.** *Ann R Col/ Surg Eng:* 78, pg 59–60.
STUDY PURPOSE Was the purpose stated clearly? ☒ Yes ☐ No	**Outline the purpose of the study. How does the study apply to your research question?** The purpose of this study was to assess the rate of UTI after short-term preoperative urethral catheterisation employing two different insertion techniques – sterile and non-sterile – and to compare costs. Since this paper looks at catheter insertion techniques its results can answer the question to my review.
LITERATURE Was relevant background literature reviewed? ☒ Yes ☐ No	**Describe the justification of the need for this study:** Very brief background; however it clearly justifies the need of the study by the statement of 'urethral catheterisation remains the most common cause of nosocomial infection in medical practice'. Statistically UTI account for 40% of all nosocomial infection all associated with indwelling catheterisation. It is clearly indicated that there are no studies investigating the effect of insertion technique priorto this Study.
DESIGN ☒ Randomized (RCT) ☐ cohort ☐ single case design ☐ before and after ☐ case-control ☐ cross-sectional ☐ case study	**Describe the study design. Was the design appropriate for the study question? (e.g., for knowledge level about this issue, outcomes, ethical issues, etc.):** The study design is a prospective Randomized Controlled design. This included all patients undergoing surgery and who needed to be catheterized: then patients were randomly allocated to one of the groups by a throw of a coin and then catheterized according to the instructions and methods used and according to the group these patients were allocated to. No indication of reason for catheterisation. **Specify any biases that may have been operating and the direction of their influence on the results:** Results could have been influenced by the type of catheter and the type of catheter coating used. The type of catheters used in this study is not stated.
SAMPLE N =156 Was the sample described in detail? ☒ Yes ☐ No	**Sampling (who;characteristics; how many; how was sampling done?) If more than one group, was there similarity between the groups?** 156 patients were included in the study, 84 females and 72 males with age range of 22 to 91 years (mean 66.8 years). The slerile technique group consisted of 74 patients with mean age of 67.5 years while the non-sterile technique group consisted of 82 patients with mean age years of 65.3 years. The authors state that there was no significant difference between groups; although the patients comprised a heterogeneous group, the two randomized

Figure 3.2 Completed McMaster University appraisal form (first page).

Data extraction

The data from the studies will be extracted and evaluated in an attempt to answer the review question; these data will be extracted by using a standardized data extraction form that was produced using the PICO framework. In this form details, facts and figures regarding study characteristics, outcome and process measures were grouped under the headings Population, Intervention and Outcomes. A copy of the data extraction form can be seen in Figure 3.3.

DATA Extraction Form

Details of Study 1:

TITLE: Randomised study of sterile versus non-sterile urethral catheterisation.
    (Authors: Carapeti EA. Andrews SM. Bentley PG.)
SOURCE: *Annals of the Royal College of Surgeons of England. 78(1):59-60, 1996 Jan.*

Reviewer's Name: Fiona Bezzina   **Date:** 6 Sept 2008

Purpose of the study: to assess the rate of UTI after short-term perioperative catheterisation using sterile versus non-sterile insertion techniques and compare the costs.

Study Design: Randomised controlled trial

POPULATION:

Sample size: 156 participants (Experimental: 82, Control: 74)

Criteria of diagnosis (CAUTI or Bacteriuria): UTI defined as Bacteriuria $> 10^5$ with or without clinical symptoms

Any Secondary diagnosis: all patients underwent surgery of some form

Inclusion / Exclusion Criteria:
    Inclusion: All surgical patients.
    Exclusion: Patients with indwelling catheters, known pre-existing UTI, those undergoing lower urinary tract surgery

Type of Catheterisation: urethral, short term, perioperative

Reason for catheterisation: Not Clear

Setting: Hospital surgical theatres

INTERVENTION:

Experimental Intervention/s: Hand washing, non-sterile gloves, tap water meatal washing, KY jelly, Catheter held in plastic sheath.
Duration of Intervention/s:
Adverse Effects: None reported

Control Treatment/s: Hand scrubbing, Gown, Sterile gloves, Sterile pack, No-touch technique, Savlon meatal cleansing, Sterile drapes, Sterile lignocaine gel, insertion with forceps
Drop-outs: None Reported

Study 1: Carapeti et al (1994):   DATA Extraction Form (Continued)

<u>**OUTCOMES:**</u>

CAUTI:

Number of UTI's (in Experimental and Control groups):

  Bacteriuria (Urine sample]: not specified
  Symptomatic UTI: not specified
  Combined Results: Experimental: 9
                          Control: 7
Types of Infecting Organisms: none specified

Time of Urine Sample / UTI (from Catheter insertion):
            First sample collected at insertion.
            Second sample 3 days post-insertion.

CAUTI Incidence Rate (as percentage) in:
            Intervention Group: 11%
            Control Group: 9.5%
            Statistical significance: P>0.1

UTI Rate according to Gender: UTI was present in 11.9% of females and in 8.3% of males
                          (P>0.1)

Figure 3.3 Data extraction form.

 Step 7: Plans for synthesizing the data (refer to Chapter 10)

Box 3.1   Checklist you can use to assess whether you have included all sections of your protocol

Title and question

- Is the title a true representation of the content?

- Are all components of the question included within the title?

- Has an appropriate question relevant to the area of expertise been developed?

Abstract

Is there a clear summary of the research, including the background, objectives (and rationale), procedures, results, conclusions and implications for the field? No more than 300–400 words.

Background

- Is the background to the area well written and would it be considered capable of promoting interest?
- Has the importance of the problem been highlighted and appropriate references used?
- Is there an explanation of how the review extends the existing literature? Or if it is a duplication of another review is it clear how the student's review is different?
- Is the relevance of the study to the field or gap in knowledge clear? That is, the student needs to show that no review exactly like theirs has been carried out.
- Does it demonstrate some knowledge of the specialist area of practice and question orthodox practice using balanced, logical and supported argument?
- Is independence of thought and open-mindedness demonstrated?

Objectives and aims

- Statement of the study's objective/s (or, if relevant, hypotheses).
- Are the objectives (or research question) based on the background?
- Is it clear how these objectives will be measured?
- Are they relevant to the clinical area under investigation?

Criteria for considering studies in review

This should follow from the research question:

- Have details of the types of participants to be included in the review been described?
- Have details been given of the types of intervention (exposure or test to be evaluated)?
- Have details been given of the types of comparative groups (or gold standard reference test) to be included in review?
- Have details been given of the types of study (designs) to be included in review?
- Have details been given of the types of outcome measures to be included in review?

Search strategy

- Are the PICOT or PEOT components of the research question identified?
- Is it clear how the student derived all the synonyms from the research question and used Boolean operators appropriately to enable the formulation of the search strategy?
- Are all databases to be searched described and the dates provided?
- Are all possible sources of literature to be searched? For example electronic databases, MEDLINE, EMBASE, PsychLIT, CINAHL, etc.?
- Are specialist trial registers checked? Cochrane?
- Is hand searching to be undertaken?
- Are reference lists to be checked?

(Continued)

Box 3.1   Continued

- Is grey literature to be checked? For example PhDs and BScs in libraries, conference proceedings or abstracts?
- Is the description of the search strategy detailed enough so that someone else could duplicate it and get the same results?
- Overall, is the search efficient and used appropriately?

Methods

Have details of all three parts of the methods section been described?

Part 1: The process of selecting papers for inclusion in the review

This process consists of two steps: the initial paper selection followed by the second, more thorough, selection of papers.

First selection of papers:

- Is the first selection of papers (for inclusion in review) based on titles and abstracts only?
- Is the student to conduct it alone or are two students to perform it independently? If alone has the student stated how this would impact the validity of the results?
- Are the procedures to be used going to be tested on a sample of articles (somewhat like a pilot study)?
- Was a standardized form made for this procedure? Is it appropriate and adequate to answer the research question?
- Was a clear description provided of the criteria the student was looking for at this stage?
- Is it clear how disagreements will be resolved (if more than one student)?

Second (more thorough) selection of papers: The criteria for this section are the same as above, except that the selection of papers is based on reading the whole paper.

Part 2: The procedure for the assessment of methodological quality

- Is the appropriate checklist used to assess the methodological quality of each paper included in the assignment? For example, if student used RCTs, controlled clinical trials (CCTs) and qualitative papers, then three checklists need to be included and described in this section.
- Are the checklists to be used well cited and referenced?
- Is it clear how many people are to assess the studies and how this is to be carried out?
- Are assessments to be done independently?
- Is a description given of how the papers are to be marked? For example, using a numerical scale or other such as very poor, poor, adequate, good, very good.

(Continued)

The data extraction strategy

* Is the appropriate data to be extracted to enable the research question to be answered?
* Is the standardized form used to extract data appropriate to collect all the data necessary to answer the research question?
* Is the data extraction form to be piloted in any way before it is used in the study?
* Is data to be extracted by one student or more than one student? Has the student discussed the implications?
* How are disagreements to be resolved (if more than one student)?

References

* Was the Harvard format used?
* Do citations and references match?
* Accurately presented?
* Wide range and scope of papers?

Presentation

* Correct layout for title page, contents, page numbers, etc.?
* Text free from errors and spelling mistakes?
* Appropriate use of vocabulary and grammar?
* Appropriate use of the appendices?
* Logical and clear presentation of appendices?
* Clear and aesthetic style and presentation of the report as a whole?

Key points

When writing your own protocol, the following key points should be considered:

* Before you start writing the full review it is important to search a number of websites where you can check if another systematic literature review of your exact review question has already been done. It would be disappointing to have done your systematic review and then find someone else conducted the same review just a few months ago.
* It is important to complete a protocol or plan for your review before starting to write the full review. This is because it enables you to:
  o identify your question
  o identify your inclusion and exclusion criteria
  o state your aims and objectives
  o clarify the criteria for selecting your studies
  o articulate the methods.

The protocol also:

    o   provides a structured and systematic approach to undertaking your review

    o   encourages the author/s to follow and not deviate from the plan

    o   identifies any potential issues before you commence your review.

- Start with the background discussion.
- Clearly state your objects (primary and secondary if needed).
- Describe the steps you plan to take to conduct your review – that is, how you will search for, select, appraise and extract data from your research papers to enable you to answer your review question.
- Be sure to include a copy of the forms to (1) select your papers, (2) assess the methodology of your included papers and (3) extract data from your papers within your protocol (they are also part of your methods).
- Finally, be sure to finish your protocol by describing how you plan to synthesize the data you extract.

Summary

This chapter has discussed the importance of writing a protocol for your systematic review and has described the steps you need to take to complete it successfully. We have also referred you to a number of websites where you can check if another systematic literature review of your exact systematic review question has already been done (see Box 1.2 in Chapter 1). A brief overview of all the steps to include within your protocol was described and an example of a real student's protocol was provided.

Question and Answer (Q&A)

(Q) What are the important messages to learn from Fay's protocol?

(A) Following a recognized framework for developing your protocol will only serve to enhance the quality and outcome of your systematic review:

- It makes undertaking and completing the review much easier.
- It helps make sure that you don't change the way you conduct the full review once you have started it.
- It reduces bias and enables replication.

References

Khan, K.S. and Zamora, J. (2022) *Systematic Reviews to Support Evidence-Based Medicine: How to Appraise, Conduct and Publish Reviews*, 3rd edn. London: Royal Society of Medicine Press.

Purssell, E. and McCrae, N. (2020) *How to Perform a Systematic Literature Review: A Guide for Healthcare Researchers, Practitioners and Students*. Cham: Springer.

University of Reading (n.d.) Doing a systematic review: Creating a protocol. Library guides. Available at https://libguides.reading.ac.uk/systematic-review/protocol (accessed 23 August 2023).

4

Writing the background to your systematic review

Overview

- The background to your systematic review
- Providing an operational definition of the clinical problem
- Highlighting the importance of the review question and grabbing the attention of the reader
- Clarifying the gap in systematic reviews in the clinical area
- Using different tools and methods to help you start writing up your background section
- The importance of managing and planning your time

The background to your systematic review

The role of the background in your protocol and subsequent systematic review is to describe the setting and context of the area of research, the importance of the topic and the reasons why it has been chosen (Greenhalgh et al. 2023; Higgins et al. 2023). There may be numerous reasons for the choice of topic, for example reporting a review to evaluate the effectiveness of a particular treatment or replicating an important systematic review in a particular area of nursing practice carried out in another country or several years previously.

A well-written background should be clear about the direction of the systematic review. In the background, it is important to explain what systematic reviews have already been conducted in this area, if any; discuss their strengths and limitations; and describe how the proposed systematic review will fill a gap in the literature, providing new information that could advance practice (Higgins et al. 2023).

The background, in addition to describing the strengths and limitations for the systematic review, should focus on the factual evidence and where possible avoid anecdotal recounting of the reasons for conducting the review. Where possible always back up your reasons with facts, figures, government/professional policy documents like those by the Nursing and Midwifery Council (NMC) and references where available. For an intervention study, the background could include some or all of the following, depending on the specific topic of your systematic review:

- Provide an operational definition of the clinical or nursing problem.
- Cite research papers or government/professional documents with statistical figures to highlight the importance of the systematic review.

- Describe the signs and symptoms (or consequences) of the disease, illness, problem or issue and its relevance to nursing.
- Provide details of the patients' age, gender and other pertinent demographic and biographic information.
- Describe the course of the disease or pathophysiology, pharmacology and other associated outcomes, such as quality of life measures, anxiety and depression scores, etc.
- If the review is related to the effectiveness of any type of intervention, there needs to be a discussion about how the disease or issue is usually managed in practice.
- Describe the general outcome measures.
- Once the problem has been discussed, including the incidence, the effects on patients' lives and management of the problem, your research should reveal an evidence or literature gap that shows why this systematic review is required. References should be provided to justify and support how your proposed systematic review is different.

Remember that you are trying to show that there is a gap in *systematic literature reviews* and not in primary research papers or narrative reviews. Some of the key issues will now be discussed individually and in more depth.

Providing an operational definition of the clinical problem

When starting the background section, it is usual to provide an operational definition of the clinical problem you are addressing in your systematic review. An operational definition is a clear, concise, detailed account of a measure, described within a particular context; here you will be stating what the problem is and what it is not. Once you have provided an operational definition and if your issue relates to a clinical problem, it is usually appropriate to describe:

- the causes of the condition
- the age of your specific population group
- the specific diagnosis
- the signs and symptoms of the illness or problem
- the natural history or course of the disease or pathophysiology.

We now provide an example of the above.

T In Tamara's example the background section on bracing and exercises for adolescents with scoliosis will require an operational definition that includes a description of the term adolescent idiopathic scoliosis (AIS) and how this leads to a clinical problem. Tamara could write something like the following:

Adolescent idiopathic scoliosis (AIS) is a deformity of the spine and rib cage which generally occurs in children and adolescents between the ages of 10 and 16 years old (SRS 2023). The causes of AIS are not known, though many theories have been put forward over the years; these include possible genetic, muscular or neurological causes, among others (SRS 2023).

As seen above, after every statement it is important to include a reference or evidence to demonstrate that this piece of information has been obtained from a reliable source. (Please note that the references used in the case extracts are for illustrative purposes only and are not included in the reference list in this book.)

Highlighting the importance of the systematic review question and grabbing the attention of the reader

There are a number of ways to clarify the importance of the systematic review question or clinical problem, including the use of statistics, key government/professional papers as well as previous important research work in the area. The use of statistics highlights the significance of the problem within the general population. For instance, the statement 'Low back pain occurs in 80 per cent of the population at some time in their lives' makes it clear that low back pain is an important clinical problem. Citing key government/professional documents within your background is a good strategy, as it demonstrates the importance that government and regulatory bodies attach to this specific area of health and/or care.

T For example, Tamara could write something like this:

> The incidence of AIS varies between different countries from 0.9 to 12 per cent (Cárcamo et al. 2023). AIS occurs much more frequently in girls and for curves of over 40 degrees and the occurrence of AIS in girls as compared with boys is approximately 8:2 or four times greater (Menger and Sin 2023).

In the example above, the statement that AIS can occur in up to 12 per cent of children, and mainly in girls, is highlighting that this is an important problem that needs to be reviewed. Once the importance of the topic has been clarified, the signs and symptoms of the clinical condition need to be discussed. In Tamara's example, she could say something like the following.

> The deformity results in a spinal curvature together with a rib hump and shoulder, waist and pelvic asymmetries (Maharathi et al. 2023). This deformity has a significant impact on these young children and adolescents. These include a decreased quality of life as well as many psychological problems such as low self-esteem and self-image (Zaina et al. 2023).

Once Tamara has discussed the clinical problem together with the resultant signs and symptoms of the condition, it is appropriate for her to describe the current management for patients with AIS, as outlined below:

> Patients with AIS are generally treated to prevent the curvature and rib hump getting any worse. The treatment type depends on the severity of the curvature and rib hump. For small curves (10–40 degrees) either annual monitoring and observation or scoliosis-specific exercises are usually recommended. Curves between 40 and 50 degrees are usually braced or observed and curves over 50 degrees are usually recommended for surgery.

Practical Tip

Detailing the background and context to your clinical problem with the backing of robust evidence is a good way of obtaining buy-in from nurse leaders, managers and commissioners to support the systematic review. Publishing your systematic review is also helpful in encouraging other student nurses, midwives and allied health professional students to undertake a systematic review.

Clarifying the gap in systematic reviews in the clinical area

Within your background, it is critical to describe and critique any previous systematic reviews that have been conducted in your specific area. You need to show that your systematic review has not been conducted recently and that yours will be the most up to date and of the highest quality. If narrative reviews have been conducted in your specific area, it is worth mentioning them and explaining that as they are narrative reviews their results may be biased. This is because in narrative reviews methodological quality is not always assessed.

If there are previous systematic reviews that you would like to include, you should provide a brief description explaining what was reviewed and when. Furthermore, you should also demonstrate how your systematic review is different from any previous ones. *Put simply, you are attempting to clarify the gap in systematic reviews in the evidence base* and to prove why your systematic review is necessary.

Note: If an identical systematic review was carried out over a year ago and no additional primary papers in this area have emerged, then it is clear that another systematic review in this area at this specific time would not be needed. This is because the evidence base has not changed.

In order for you to show the gap in systematic reviews in your specific area, you need to describe what other reviews have been conducted, whether they were narrative or systematic reviews, how long ago they were conducted, and to what extent your proposed systematic review is similar and, more importantly, to what extent it is different.

T Returning to Tamara's example, at the end of the extract below she quotes from work by Negrini et al. (2015):

To date, reviews in this area have been mostly narrative reviews that have not included the evaluation of the methodological quality of the included studies and relevant primary papers. For example, the narrative review by [name of researcher] (year of publication) did not include all primary papers in the area and

the narrative review by [name of researcher] (year of publication) did not evaluate the methodological quality of the included primary papers. One systematic
review was found, but this related to the effect of braces on adults and not adolescents with idiopathic scoliosis. A 'gold standard' systematic review is needed to
make sure that the 'sacrifices that children are making when wearing a brace are
indeed worthwhile' (Negrini et al. 2015).

Should you wish to read the whole background of this review you can find the
details in the list of references of this chapter.

Tamara's examples are based on the original (2010) and updated (2015) systematic reviews, but we would like to clarify that we have omitted some authors and/or
added or changed a few sentences in order to provide an illustration of how the text
could be written in your own systematic review and show how to make a point or
present an argument.

Using different tools and methods to help you start writing up your background section

Several tools are available for you to access and apply in order to help you write up
the background section to your systematic review. These include, but are not limited
to, some of the following:

- **Nursing concept maps**:
  Nursing concept mapping is a graphical tool for defining patient issues, organizing
  assessment results, selecting relevant diagnoses and procedures, and assessing
  outcomes. Nurses, midwives and AHP students can effectively and efficiently
  devise strategies using the services and tools of this concept map. (Nursing
  Concept Maps n.d.)
- **Patient journey mapping:** This is a rapidly growing approach for better
  understanding how people enter, experience, and exit health services. This type of
  methodology has significant potential to inform new, patient centered models
  of care and facilitate nurses, midwives, patients and other health and care professionals to better understand gaps and strategies in care services (Davies et al.
  2023). The usefulness of mind mapping in nursing care is in highlighting how
  effective nursing is in engaging with patients and family members in meeting their
  needs (Ruppel et al. 2023).
- **Mind mapping in nursing:**
  Mind mapping uses a technique of combining drawings with words to build
  memory links between a topic keyword and image, color, or other link, thereby
  highlighting the key point and level of the memory contents, allowing learners to
  effectively store and extract information. Mind mapping is a sound training tool
  in thinking that not only improves learning efficiency but also increases learning
  motivation and interest. (Wu and Wu 2020)
- **Idea generation in nursing**: Idea generation in nursing is linked to creativity,
  and is often associated with the generation of ideas or products that are original and useful to enhancing nursing care and practice. Creativity consists of two

important concepts, aligned to divergent and convergent thinking. Divergent thinking is the ability to generate ideas and convergent thinking is vital for the evaluation and selection of the most promising options for implementation. To be creative, one has to be able to switch between these two modes of thinking (Ritter and Mostert 2018). Brainstorming, detailed below, is a method of idea generation in nursing.

In Tamara's case study, she is aware that if she begins writing too early she may be forced to stop and go back to the initial steps because the activities outlined in Box 4.1 were not entirely completed. Once these steps have been completed, Tamara can feel confident that she has searched widely and has read a number of review papers, government documents and research papers in the general area of AIS, braces and scoliosis-specific exercises. She has also been trying to identify what is known and what is not known about her systematic review question. She will begin to write her background only when she is confident that she can answer 'Yes' to the six questions listed in Box 4.1. We recommend that you too complete Box 4.1 for your own systematic review.

Box 4.1   Template to complete for your background section

1. Have you searched and read broadly in the area of your specific review question?   YES ☐   NO ☐

2. Have you made sure that a number of primary research papers have been conducted relating to your specific area of interest? *(It does not matter if there are no primary papers available. This only reaffirms the need for your systematic review. This means that your systematic review may possibly be an 'empty' review.)*   YES ☐   NO ☐

3. Have you spent time thinking critically about your specific review topic?   YES ☐   NO ☐

4. Have you spent time discussing your review topic with your colleagues or supervisor with a knowledge of this area?   YES ☐   NO ☐

5. Have you found out how people in other disciplines think about your research topic?   YES ☐   NO ☐

6. Do you feel ready to begin writing your research protocol?   YES ☐   NO ☐

Having completed Box 4.1, provided you have answered yes to all questions, you can now begin to think about and work up the content of the background section for your systematic review. Some student nurses and midwives undertaking a systematic review in nursing for the first time may be unsure about how and where to start. A way around this is to engage with and use any of the different mind mapping tools mentioned above, such as concept mapping, journey mapping, mind mapping and idea generation. Any of these mind mapping tools will enable you to:

- represent ideas, thoughts and feelings as 'concepts' or 'knowledge structures' used in learning, in a two-dimensional graphic arrangement.
- label and link concepts to form linear associations or hierarchies.

The center represents the hub or central theme from where the various 'roads' on the map emerge. By presenting ideas in a radial, graphical, linear or non-linear manner, mind maps encourage a brainstorming approach to planning and organizing tasks which illustrate the various components of your background contained within your systematic review.

Mind mapping enables brainstorming which, in our opinion, is a highly creative technique in which an individual or group of people try to establish the facts and/or a solution for a specific problem. This is achieved by gathering a list of ideas spontaneously contributed by the participant/s. Although Tamara could do this activity on her own, she decides to get together with a group of her colleagues. This is important, as they may have ideas and thoughts about the topic that she may not have thought about prior to beginning to draw a mind map on the topic of braces and scoliosis-specific exercises for adolescents with scoliosis. We would suggest you draw and illustrate your mind map in Box 4.2 below.

Box 4.2   Your initial brainstorming mind map

Try to make a mind map for your own systematic review question.

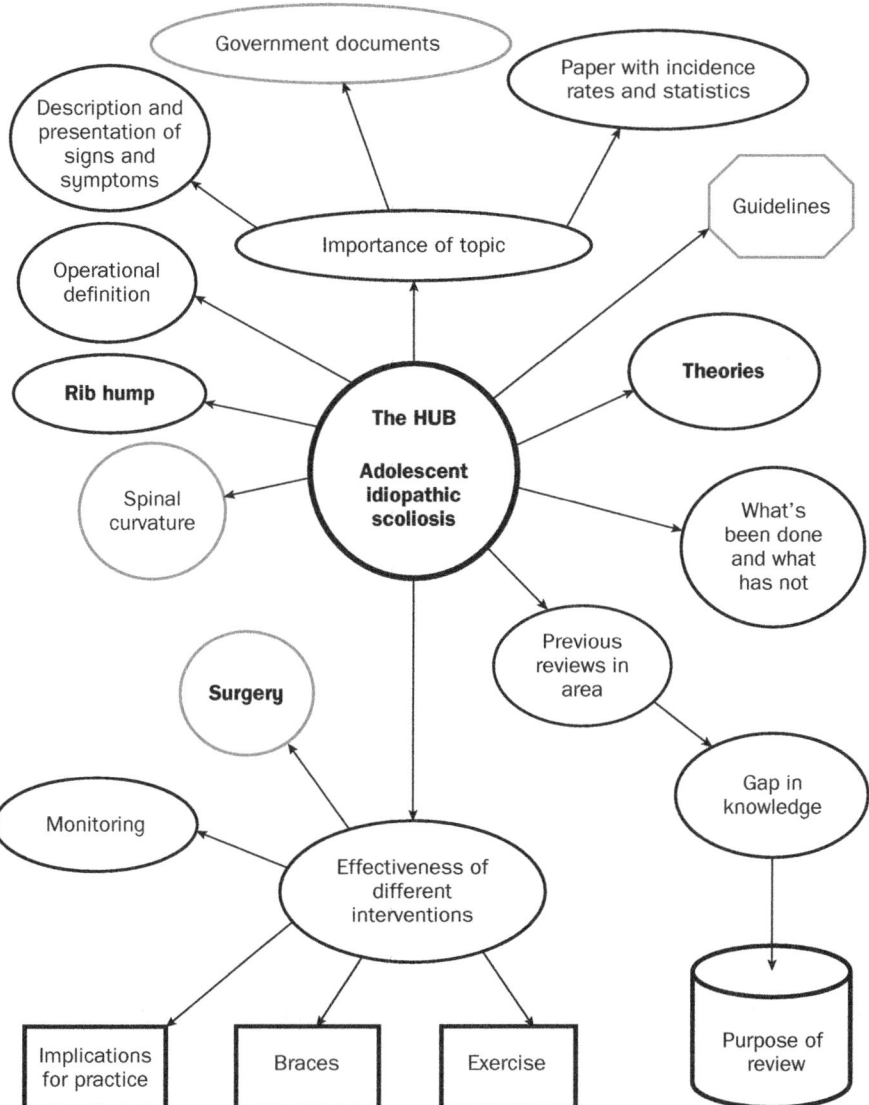

T **Figure 4.1** Example of a mind map that Tamara could make on her topic of braces and exercises for scoliosis.

An example of Tamara's initial brainstorming mind map is provided in Figure 4.1, followed by the completed and ordered mind map in Figure 4.2.

Box 4.3 should be used to organize your mind map in the order in which you plan to write it in the background.

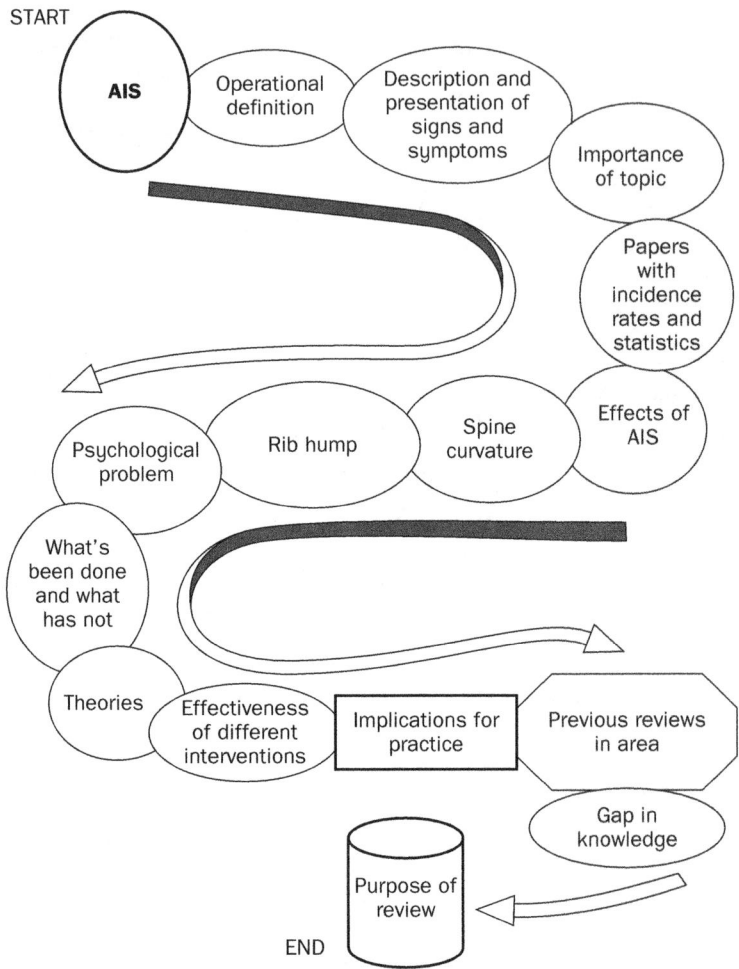

T **Figure 4.2** Tamara organizes her mind map in the order in which she plans to write it up.

Practical Tip

As identified above there are numerous software packages available that can help you to develop your own ideas and mind maps. In some instances, these can be obtained free online, and can help support you in presenting your ideas/findings in a visual way. Before you begin mind mapping ensure you familiarize yourself with the software; it will save you time later.

Box 4.3   Your mind map in the order that you plan to write it out

---

If you are unable to access any of the various mind mapping tools, all is not lost. There are still ways of developing your ideas and background, as demonstrated in the next section.

Alternative types of templates

If you prefer, you can use a list instead of a mind map to write the topics that you would like to include in your background. Start by listing each issue, one beneath the other, in the same order that you plan to write them up in your own background. Provide plenty of space to capture your ideas, thoughts and feelings. Referring to Tamara's case study, an example is detailed in Table 4.1. This list is not exhaustive.

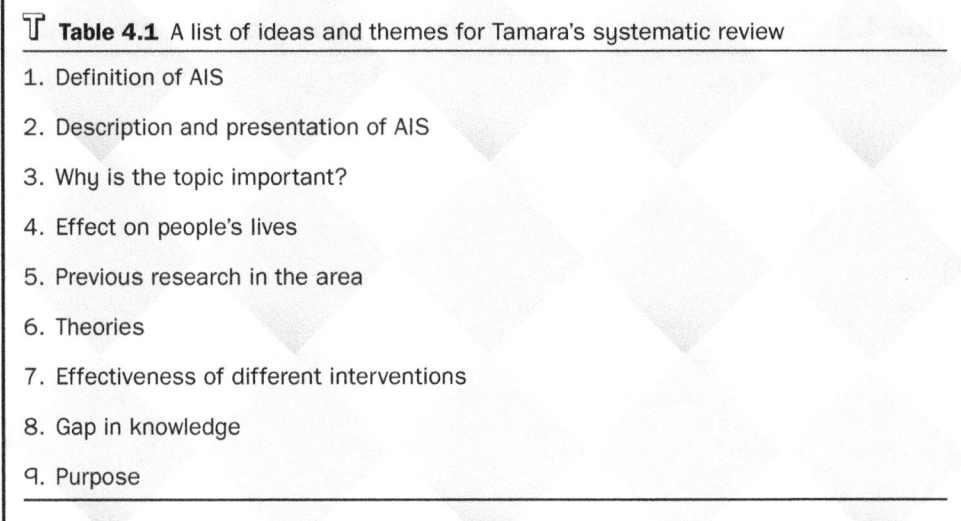

Table 4.1 A list of ideas and themes for Tamara's systematic review

1. Definition of AIS

2. Description and presentation of AIS

3. Why is the topic important?

4. Effect on people's lives

5. Previous research in the area

6. Theories

7. Effectiveness of different interventions

8. Gap in knowledge

9. Purpose

Box 4.4 is a template for you to list all the points for your own background.

Box 4.4   Template for listing the points for your own background
1
2
4
4
5
6
7
8
9

Once Tamara has made a list of all the concepts, she decides to add another column to her list. In this column she writes all the possible sources of information that she may require and makes sure that they are available nearby so she can refer to them as she writes. Building on Table 4.1, Table 4.2 shows Tamara's new list, which comprises both ideas and themes along with possible sources of information. Box 4.5 provides a template for you to list your own themes and possible sources of information for your own systematic review.

Table 4.2 Tamara's themes and possible sources of information

	Themes	Possible sources of information and activities to do
1.	Definition of AIS	Dictionary Government documents Review documents Research papers
2.	Description and presentation	As above
43	Importance of topic	Papers with statistics and incidence rates Government health department documents
4.	Effect on people's lives	All above, especially research papers and reviews
5.	Previous research in area	Research papers and systematic reviews or other reviews in a similar or related area
6.	Theories	Theoretical papers or research papers primarily
7.	Effectiveness of different interventions	Research papers showing effectiveness of different intervention studies
8.	Gap in knowledge	All above, highlighting what has and has not been done yet
9.	Purpose	This will address the gap above

Having identified and discussed Tamara's case study background, we will now provide a commentary on Fay's background on urinary tract infections. Please note that the references within Fay's extracts are used for illustrative purposes only and are therefore not included within the book.

F Commentary on Fay's background section

To go back to what was said above on pages 86 and 87 of this chapter, these are some of the points that could be included in your background section, especially if you are conducting a systematic review on an intervention. In the following pages you will find a few excerpts from Fay's background section; next to each excerpt is the point (or number) that it is addressing. We would suggest you refer to the protocol in Chapter 3 to remind yourself of where these excerpts 'sit' within the background section. So, to repeat what we said on pages 57 and 58 of this chapter, your background could include some or all of the following, depending on the specific topic of your review:

1 Provide an operational definition of the clinical problem.

2 Cite research papers or government documents with statistical figures to highlight the importance of the study.

Box 4.5   Template for listing your own themes and possible sources of information

	Themes	Possible sources of information
1	Operational definition	
2		
3		
4		
5		
6		
7		
8		
9		

③ Describe the signs and symptoms (or consequences) of the disease, illness, problem or issue.

④ Provide details of the patients' age, gender and other pertinent details.

⑤ Describe the course of the disease or pathophysiology.

⑥ If the review is related to the effectiveness of any type of intervention, there needs to be a discussion about how the disease or issue is usually managed in practice.

⑦ Describe the general outcome measures.

⑧ Once the problem has been discussed, including incidence, effect on patients' lives and management, *a gap in systematic reviews in the evidence or literature needs to be identified.*
References should be used to support how the proposed review is different from other systematic reviews in the area.

Below you will find excerpts from Fay's background section; her proposal can be found in Chapter 3 on pages 62–80. Please note that the number icons within the boxes refer to the number of the point in the list above that the excerpt is addressing.

Example 1

> ① *Hospital-acquired infection can be defined as an infection that is neither present nor incubating at the time of admission to hospital (Hospital Acquired Infection [online]).*

Commentary: Fay starts by offering a general operational definition of what hospital acquired infection is. (This is a definition that explains 'what something is' within the context in which you are using it; this is very important to state in order to ensure that all readers of your work understand specifically what you are talking about.) Later, she focuses this to define what catheter-associated urinary tract infection (CAUTI) is in practice. It is a good idea to provide a definition(s) of your clinical area of concern as soon as possible in the background (point 1 above).

Example 2

> ② *Urinary catheterization of patients is a common nursing procedure used both in the hospital and in the community. According to Dougherty and Lister (2004, pg 444) catheter-associated infections are the most common nosocomial infection, accounting for up to around 45% of all hospital-acquired infections.*

Commentary: Fay starts her background by showing us the importance of her topic and letting the reader know that CAUTIs are very common. She also strengthens her statement by letting us know that they make up 45 per cent of hospital-acquired infections and backs this up using a reference (point 2 above).

Example 3

> 2 *Studies by Bryan and Reynolds (1984, pg 494–498) and Turck and Stamm (1981, pg 651–654) concluded that between 75% and 80% of all healthcare-associated UTIs follow the insertion of a urinary catheter, and a study by Glynn et al. (1997), which investigated 40 English hospitals, estimated that around 26% of all hospitalized patients have a urinary catheter inserted, whilst Parker (1999, pg 564–574) and Godfrey and Evans (2000, pg 682– 690) suggest that 4% of patients in the community, at some point, will have a catheter inserted.*

Commentary: Fay goes a step further here and provides the statistics and references to show that up to 80 per cent of healthcare UTIs follow the insertion of a urinary catheter. This statement suggests (to some degree at least) that had the catheter not been inserted or had further care or a more sterile environment been used, these infections may have been prevented. In other words, Fay is further highlighting the importance of this issue to healthcare both in hospitals as well as in the community.

Example 4

> 3, 2 & 5 *Furthermore, complications that may arise from urinary catheterization include structural damage to the urinary tract, bleeding, false passage and urinary tract infections and bacteriuria (Joanna Briggs online).*

Commentary: By describing all the complications (point 3) that can arise from the insertion of a catheter, Fay is again highlighting the importance of her research question within the area of healthcare (point 2). She is also describing the course of the disease or pathophysiology (point 5).

Example 5

> 2 *It is estimated that CAUTI costs the National Health Service (NHS) £1,427 per patient and because it increases the period of hospitalization of such patients by approximately three to six days, costs approximately increase by £124 million per year (Hart, 2008, pg 44–48; SSHAIP, 2004, [online]).*

Commentary: By providing the actual figures for the increased costs that CAUTI can result in, Fay is again highlighting the importance of this clinical problem and suggesting that this issue needs to be looked at urgently. Detailing this information may help Fay receive support from nurse leaders, managers and commissioners to do the review.

Example 6

> 1 *A catheter is a tubular device which is passed through the urethra into the bladder in order to drain urine or to instill medical treatment (Dougherty and Lister, 2004, pg 440–444; Steward, in BJN monograph, 2001, pg 42).*

Commentary: Here Fay is providing the reader with the operational definitions of what a catheter is and when it should be used. As discussed above, an operational definition is a definition that explains 'what something is' within the context in which you are using it. Operational definitions are very important, as they help ensure that all readers of your work understand specifically what you are talking about. In other words, to use very colloquial terminology, they help to make sure that 'everyone is singing from the same hymn sheet'.

Example 7

> 6 *Catheterization is indicated in and used to relieve obstructed flow of urine, to measure the residual amount in the bladder, to provide post-operative drainage following bladder, vaginal and prostate surgery, in monitoring hourly urine output in the critically ill patient, and in continence care (Brunner and Suddarth, 1992, pg 682; Steward, in BJN monograph, 2001, pg 42). Insertion of a urinary catheter is a common procedure in both acute and primary care settings, and careful consideration is always required over the need for versus the risk of this procedure.*

Commentary: Here Fay is describing when and why catheterization is used – again to clarify for the reader the situations when it is needed. You will note that she mentions that 'careful' consideration is always required over the need for versus the risk of this procedure, as complications and infections are so common (as she mentioned above).

Example 8

> 6 & 2 *Urethral catheterization may be performed as an indwelling or an intermittent procedure. Indwelling catheterization consists of continuous catheter drainage which can be sub-classified into short term (1–7 days), mid term (7–28 days) and long term (28 days up to 4 months) (Hart, 2008,*

> *pg 44–48; Head, 2006, pg 44–46; RCN, 2008, pg 2–55). Intermittent catheterization consists of episodic introduction of a catheter into the bladder to drain urine out (Dougherty and Lister, 2004, pg 445). The catheter is passed via the urethra and removed soon after the bladder urine is drained. In recent years this technique has become noticeably popular, and can be carried out by the patient him/herself or by the nurse. This form of catheterization is indicated for the drainage of a poorly functioning bladder (as is found in spinal cord injury patients and those with neurological disorders) and for the urinary drainage in the peri-operative period. Its main advantage is that the patient is left catheter-free in between catheterizations (Dougherty and Lister, 2004, pg 445; Robinson, 2007, pg 48–56). Intermittent catheterization is also commonly used to instill medications, measure residual urine, and it is also used to instill contrast material into the bladder to study the bladder and the urethra (Hart, 2008, pg 44–48). Lapides et al. (2002, pg 1584–1586) and Wilson (1998, pg S10–14) advocate that this procedure should be undertaken as a sterile procedure in the hospital environment due to the high risk of hospital-acquired infections, while in the community a clean technique should be used.*

Commentary: Fay is now describing the different types of catheterization (in other words the different types of the intervention that are available and how the intervention is applied) (point 6). She is also using numerous references to support her statements (point 2).

Example 9

> 5 *CAUTI is asymptomatic in the majority of cases (Tambyah et al., 2000, pg 678–682); however, Godfrey and Evans (2000, pg 682–690) clarify that CAUTI can present with signs and symptoms such as: pyrexia, pyuria, urinary bypassing of the catheter, cloudy foul-smelling urine, confusion in elderly patients, haematuria and back pain.*

Commentary: Fay clearly defines what CAUTI is and the associated signs and symptoms.

Example 10

> 4 *These symptoms may vary with the age and sex of the patient and also with the severity and site of the infection. Pickerman (1994, pg 66–68) suggests that these signs and symptoms occur when the bacteria invade the bladder mucosa resulting in inflammation. Diagnosis is established after obtaining a urine sample for culture and sensitivity.*

Commentary: Fay makes it clear that the signs and symptoms may vary with age, gender and location of the infection. She also makes it clear how the diagnosis is obtained.

Example 11

> ⑦ *A bacterial count of 100,000 organisms (or CFU) per millilitre is considered to be significant of urinary tract infection. Bacteriuria and urinary tract infection are two terms used interchangeably in the nursing literature. Bacteriuria is the presence of bacteria in the urine; however, according to Higgins (1995, pg 44–45) bacteriuria in patients with indwelling and intermittent catheters does not always suggest a diagnosis of urinary tract infection (UTI).*

Commentary: In this paragraph Fay describes what exactly constitutes a significant bacterial infection and how this may present itself clinically. Fay also describes how this outcome is measured objectively per millilitre – that is, a bacterial count of 100,000 organisms (or CFU) per millilitre.

Example 12

> ⑧ *Three systematic reviews were identified in the literature. The review by Jamison et al. (2004) focuses mainly on the use of catheter types in management of the neurogenic bladder whereas the review by Niel-Weise and Van den Broek (2005) looked at studies comparing urethral indwelling, intermittent and suprapubic catheterization. The review by Lockwood et al. (2004, pg 271–291) treated the issue of sterility at insertion very briefly; only two relevant studies were included. Since these reviews focused mainly on other catheter-related matters, their search strategy, therefore, could have resulted in studies relevant to the antiseptic issue being missed and left out. This study focused solely on this particular issue of sterility at catheter insertion and adopted a search strategy that would include as many of the studies that specifically dealt with this topic.*

Commentary: This highlights the importance of identifying a knowledge deficit (gap) within existing systematic reviews. This is imperative because it highlights the importance of your systematic review within the existing evidence base.

The importance of managing and planning your time

Irrespective of whether you are conducting a systematic review for an academic course or a professional qualification, or even as part of a research project, it is a time-consuming process. It is therefore vital that you set aside enough time to undertake and complete it successfully. A couple of practical things to remember are as follows:

- **Academic and professional courses and programmes**: If you are writing a systematic review dissertation or have to undertake a systematic review for a module or a professional course or programme, you will have been given specific criteria to write this. You will therefore need a significant period of time (perhaps 4–6 months) depending on how much time you can devote to undertaking and writing it up.

- **Continuing professional development:** If you are conducting a systematic review as part of your continuing professional development or for a commissioned piece of work, or even if you are completing it as part of a Cochrane or Campbell review, we suggest that you should set aside at least 6–12 months just to write your protocol. You will then need possibly another 12 months to undertake the review, complete the review processes and write it up.

- **Activities and timetabling:** We usually recommend to our students to make a timetable of all the activities involved and to set a deadline for each activity. Developing a Gantt chart is a good way of illustrating the planned activities to be completed over time. A Gantt chart contains a series of horizontal lines showing the type and amount of work to be produced and completed within a certain period of time. The value of Gantt charts for conducting your systematic review is in the way they illustrate the start and finish dates of all elements contained within your review. An example of a Gantt chart is shown in Table 4.3. Box 4.6 is provided

Table 4.3 Example of a Gantt chart

	Weeks or months	1	2	3	4	5	6	7	8	9
Activities		▓	▓							
Select an area and carry out background reading		▓	▓							
Develop a question			▓	▓						
Write the background				▓	▓					
Write the objectives						▓				
Write the criteria						▓				
Select your studies							▓			
Appraise your studies							▓	▓		
Extract data								▓		
Write results								▓	▓	
Write discussion									▓	▓
Write up paper or dissertation										▓

Box 4.6   Template Gantt chart for your own systematic review

Weeks or months	1	2	3	4	5	6	7	8	9
Activities									
Select an area and carry out background reading									
Develop a question									
Write the background									
Write the objectives									
Write the criteria									
Select your studies									
Appraise your studies									
Extract data									
Write results									
Write discussion									
Write up paper or dissertation									

for you to use for your own systematic review; you may want to change the word 'weeks' to 'months', etc. A useful article by Fontaine et al. (2022), titled 'Designing, planning, and conducting systematic reviews and other knowledge syntheses: six key practical recommendations to improve feasibility and efficiency', offers some useful and practical tips for organizing a good systematic review.

> ### Practical Tip
>
> If you can demonstrate that your potential systematic review is linked to address-ing and/or resolving an existing clinical problem/need in your area of work, you may be able to use this as leverage to negotiate with your nurse leaders, manag-ers and/or commissioners for some time off to undertake and complete the review.

Key points

- Writing a protocol of what you intend to include before you start your system-atic review is very important.
- A protocol describes, in advance, the systematic review question together with your background and rationale for the methods that you plan to use. It also includes details of how different types of studies will be located, appraised and synthesized.
- Once you have formulated your systematic review question, it is a good idea to undertake a quick general search (also called a scoping search) to make sure that there are no systematic literature reviews already available or in progress that address your exact systematic review question.
- A protocol includes all of the following sections:
  - An answerable, systematic review question
  - The background to the review
  - The objectives of the review
  - The inclusion and exclusion criteria
  - The search strategy
  - The proposed methods for selecting, appraising and extracting the rel-evant data from the chosen research papers to answer your systematic review question.
- The background in the protocol (and later in the review) describes the setting and context of the area of research, the importance of the topic and the rea-sons why it has been chosen. In the background section of your protocol, you may consider including some of the following:
  - Provide an operational definition of the clinical problem.
  - Cite research papers or government documents with statistical figures to highlight the importance of the study.

- Describe the signs and symptoms of the disease.
- Provide details of the patients' age, gender and other pertinent information.
- Describe the course of the disease.
- If the review is related to the effectiveness of any type of intervention, there needs to be a discussion about how the disease or issue is usually managed in practice.
- Describe the general outcome measures.
- Identify a systematic review gap in the evidence or literature.
- Use references to support how the proposed review is different.
- There are a number of different tools, such as mind maps and lists, that you can use to help you write up the background section of your review.
- Gantt charts are a useful medium to help you plan and manage your workload in a timely and orderly manner.

Summary

This chapter has discussed the key factors that need to be considered when writing a protocol for your systematic literature review. The different sections within the protocol were described and examples provided. The first stage of the protocol, the background, was detailed and excerpts were included to clarify this process. Different tools and methods were suggested to help you start writing up the background section of your protocol and to manage your workload in a timely and effective manner.

Question and Answer (Q&A)

(Q) Why is writing the background section to the systematic review so time-consuming?

(A) Taking the time to research and detail the background and context regarding why your systematic review is important will have a huge impact on the outcome of the final systematic review. For example, it takes time to obtain, review, collate and synthesize policy documents, recent evidence, statistics, facts and figures.

Taking the time to develop a robust background will also help you to highlight to nurse leaders, managers and commissioners why the systematic review is needed. It may help you secure financial backing and support (in the form of time off) to undertake the systematic review.

References

Davies, E.L., Bulto, L.N., Walsh, A. et al. (2023) Reporting and conducting patient journey mapping research in healthcare: A scoping review. *Journal of Advanced Nursing* 79: 83–100.

Fontaine, G., Maheu-Cadotte, M.-A., Lavallée, A. et al. (2022) Designing, planning, and conducting systematic reviews and other knowledge syntheses: Six key practical recommendations to improve feasibility and efficiency. *Worldviews on Evidence-Based Nursing* 19: 434–441.

Greenhalgh, T.M., Bidewell, J., Crisp, E. and Warland, J. (2023) *Understanding Research Methods for Evidence-Based Practice in Health*, 3rd edn. London: John Wiley and Sons.

Higgins, J.P.T., Thomas, J., Chandler, J., Cumpston, M. et al. (eds) (2023) *Cochrane Handbook for Systematic Reviews of Interventions*, version 6.4 (updated August 2023). Available at www. training.cochrane.org/handbook (accessed 31 August 2023).

Negrini, S., Minozzi, S., Bettany-Saltikov, J. et al. (2015) Braces for idiopathic scoliosis in adolescents. Cochrane Database of Systematic Reviews 6, Art. no. CD006850. Available at https:// www.cochranelibrary.com/cdsr/doi/10.1002/14651858.CD006850.pub3/epdf/full (accessed 4 April 2024).

Nursing Content Maps (n.d.) Nursing concept maps examples: Do you know the types of nursing concept maps? Available at https://www.edrawmind.com/article/nursing-concept-map-examples.html#:~:text=Nursing%20concept%20mapping%20is%20a,tools%20of%20this%20 concept%20map (accessed 7 September 2023).

Ritter S. and Mostert, N.M. (2018) How to facilitate a brainstorming session: The effect of idea generation techniques and of group brainstorm after individual brainstorm. *Creative Industries Journal* 11 (3): 263–277.

Ruppel, H., McCabe, M., Tickner, M. et al. (2023) Developing a nursing dashboard to align nursing care delivery with patient and family needs. *Journal of Nursing Administration* 53 (4): 197–203.

Wu, H.Z. and Wu, Q.T. (2020) Impact of mind mapping on the critical thinking ability of clinical nursing students and teaching application. *Journal of International Medical Research* 48 (3): 300060519893225.

5

Specifying your objectives and inclusion and exclusion criteria

Overview

- Clarifying the preliminaries: problem statement, review question, aims and objectives
- Stating your aims and objectives
- Issues to consider when writing your problem statement, aims, objectives, review question and title
- Specifying the inclusion and exclusion criteria for selecting primary research papers

Clarifying the preliminaries: Problem statement, review question, aims and objectives

To avoid making mistakes when undertaking a systematic review, it is important to be clear with regards to the precise meaning and the differences between a problem statement, a review question, as well as aims and objectives. Depending on which papers or books you read, these terms may sometimes be used interchangeably. This occurs quite frequently with the terms 'objectives' and 'aims', which have slightly different meanings.

A *problem statement* is a simple statement of 'what is'. For example: 'It is not known if treatment 1 or treatment 2 is more effective for treating adult patients with chronic obstructive pulmonary disease (COPD).' A problem statement means that you are simply *stating* a problem.

The *systematic review question* follows on from the problem and the problem statement. This involves changing the problem statement into a systematic review question (detailed in Chapter 2). Consider this problem statement: 'It is not known if treatment 1 (stopping smoking) or treatment 2 (physiotherapy breathing and exercise activities) is more effective for treating adult patients with COPD.' To change this statement into a systematic review question, all you need to do is rephrase it into a question like this: 'Is treatment 1 or treatment 2 more effective in treating adult patients with COPD?' The easiest way to do this is to use similar or even identical terminology, to ensure that there is no change in meaning between the problem statement and the systematic review question.

Once you have written the systematic review question, how are the aims and objectives derived? In most dictionaries you will find that the terms 'aim' and 'objective' are synonymous (that is, words meaning the same thing), with both terms referring to the purpose for doing something. Within the area of systematic reviews, these terms tend to be used for describing the various types of research aligned to your systematic review– that is, quantitative, qualitative and mixed methods.

What is the difference between the aims and the objectives in a systematic review? The term 'aim' is usually used to state the overall purpose and goal of your systematic review, which originate from within the background and context section of your review. The aim needs to be clearly detailed whether your review is a qualitative, quantitative and/or mixed-methods systematic review. In contrast, objectives are specific statements describing the various activities and actions required by you to achieve the aim. Objectives provide the road map for undertaking the systematic review, help to clarify the review question and ensure that you stay focused, on track and on time.

Generally speaking, the 'aim' of a project is to solve the problem and answer the question, and it is usually a general statement (Jenkins et al. 1998; Davies 2019), whereas the term 'objective' is more specific. The objectives usually state what the researcher (you) are going to do to achieve the aim. For every aim, there are usually two or more objectives. In the example above, 'Is treatment 1 or treatment 2 more effective in treating adult patients with COPD?', there are a number of activities that you will need to do to achieve your aims and objectives. Box 5.1 details an example of how you could present your problem statement, systematic review question, aim, objectives and systematic review title.

Box 5.1   Example relating to the effectiveness of treatments for patients with COPD

Problem statement
It is not known if treatment 1 or treatment 2 is more effective for treating patients with COPD.

Review question
Is treatment 1 (stopping smoking) or treatment 2 (physiotherapy breathing and exercise activities) more effective for treating patients with COPD?

Aim
The aim of this study is to evaluate if there is a difference between treatment 1 and treatment 2 for patients with COPD.

Objectives
To achieve the aim the researcher will

- collect data on the effectiveness of treatment 1 and treatment 2
- compare the effectiveness of the two treatments
- synthesize the findings from the two treatments
- compare the final findings of this study with other studies
- provide recommendations/guidelines for helping patients with COPD.

Title of review
A systematic literature review comparing the effectiveness of treatment 1 and treatment 2 for treating patients with COPD.

An additional example is provided in Box 5.2, for Tamara's case study.

T Box 5.2   Tamara's example relating to the effectiveness of treatments for adolescent patients with scoliosis

Problem statement
It is not known if treatment 1 (bracing) or treatment 2 (exercise) is more effective for treating adolescent patients with scoliosis.

Review question
Is treatment 1 or treatment 2 more effective for treating adolescent patients with scoliosis?

Aim
The aim of this systematic review is to evaluate if there is a difference between the effectiveness of treatment 1 and that of treatment 2 for adolescent patients with scoliosis.

Objectives
- Collect data on the effectiveness of treatment 1 and treatment 2.
- Compare the effectiveness of the two treatments.
- Synthesize the findings from the two treatments.
- Compare the findings of this study with other studies.
- Provide guidelines for helping adolescent patients with scoliosis.

Title of review
Comparing the effectiveness of bracing to that of scoliosis exercises for treating adolescent patients with scoliosis: A systematic review.

Stating your aims and objectives

Practical Tip

Remember: the 'aim' is to write a general statement outlining the problem and the 'objective' is a series of statements about how you intend to achieve your aim. This can only be achieved by planning and managing all the activities required to address the problem. It is important that you think in terms of what you are going to be doing and how this will help you to complete the systematic review.

Once you have written a draft of the background (detailed in Chapter 4) for your systematic review, you will need to state the aim or aims and the objectives for your systematic review. It is important that the aims and objectives include all the PICOT (population, intervention, comparative intervention, outcomes and types of studies) or PEOT (population, exposure, outcomes and types of studies) elements, as detailed in Chapter 2.

T Let's refer back to Tamara's question: 'In patients with adolescent idiopathic scoliosis how effective is spinal bracing as compared with other treatments at reducing spinal curvature, rib hump and psychological problems?' Tamara's aim is to solve this problem and answer the question. Tamara's aim becomes: 'The aim of this review is to evaluate the effectiveness of spinal bracing and scoliosis-specific exercises as compared with other treatments at reducing spinal curvature, rib hump and psychological problems.' The main difference between the review question and the aim is that the former is a question and the latter is a statement. Before Tamara writes her objectives, she needs to consider what she will need to do in order to conduct her systematic review. Tamara's objectives could be, for example:

- Search for papers on the effectiveness of braces and scoliosis-specific exercises.
- Collect data on the effectiveness of braces and scoliosis-specific exercises and all other treatments.
- Compare primary papers on the effectiveness of the treatments above.
- Compare the findings of this systematic review with other reviews.
- Provide guidelines on the effectiveness of braces and scoliosis-specific exercises for helping adolescent patients with scoliosis.

Case studies

The case studies for Sue and Mary are introduced below.

S Case study: Sue, an intensive care nurse

Sue is an experienced qualified nurse working in an intensive care unit. She has seen a number of patients who have been brought into accident and emergency (A&E) following severe car accidents and have been resuscitated. She has witnessed the grief that relatives experienced, which was exacerbated when they had not been allowed to be with their loved ones during this traumatic event. This was made worse if their loved one died and they had not been present during the attempted resuscitation. Sue decided to conduct a systematic review on this subject as part of her continuing professional development.

M Case study: Mary, an A&E nurse

Mary is a newly qualified nurse working in A&E who often sees women who have been physically abused and brought in with severe facial and body bruises. This has led her to become interested in the area of domestic violence. Her review question is: 'For women who have experienced domestic violence, how effective are advocacy programmes as compared with routine treatments (usually there are no routine treatments) in terms of women's quality of life (as measured by a specific validated scale)?'

M Mary's aim will be similar to her question, for example: 'The aim of this review is to evaluate the effectiveness of advocacy programmes as compared with other treatments in terms of the quality of life of women victims of domestic violence.' As you can see in both the question and the aim, Mary has stated the population, the intervention, the comparative intervention and the outcomes. The next step is for her to write out her objectives. Like Tamara, Sue and Mary need to consider all the activities they will be doing to conduct their systematic literature reviews, so Mary's objectives could be as follows:

- Search for papers on the effectiveness of advocacy programmes and other treatments.
- Collect data on the effectiveness of advocacy programmes and other treatments.
- Compare primary papers on the different treatments (e.g. advocacy versus no advocacy).
- Compare the findings of this systematic review with other systematic reviews. (If there are no other systematic reviews in this area then you can compare it to narrative reviews.)
- Provide guidelines for helping women victims of domestic violence.

Issues to consider when writing your problem statement, aims, objectives, review question and title

It is important when writing your review to ensure that you always use the same words when writing out the title, the problem statement, the review question, the aim and the objectives. Using different words for your PICOT elements in all of the above may result in different meanings. A common mistake among student nurses we have taught is that they have used different terms when writing out each of the above, resulting in the title and aims being different. You will notice in the two examples in Tables 5.1 and 5.2 that the same words are used throughout. Box 5.3 on page 115 provides a template for recording your own problem statement, review question, aim, objectives and title for your systematic review.

M **Table 5.1** Mary's systematic review on domestic violence (quantitative review)

Problem statement	Little is known on the effectiveness of advocacy programmes as compared with other treatments in terms of women's quality of life for women who have experienced domestic violence.
Review question	For women who have experienced domestic violence, how effective are advocacy programmes as compared with other treatments in terms of women's quality of life?
Aim	The aim of this study is to evaluate the effectiveness of advocacy programmes as compared with other treatments in terms of women's quality of life for women who have experienced domestic violence.

(continued)

Ⓜ **Table 5.1** continued

Objectives	• Search for papers on the effectiveness of advocacy programmes and other treatments.
	• Collect data on the effectiveness of advocacy programmes and other treatments.
	• Compare the primary papers related to the different treatments.
	• Compare the findings of this systematic review with the findings from other systematic reviews.
	• Provide practical guidelines for helping women who have experienced or are experiencing domestic violence.
Title	A systematic literature review on the effectiveness of advocacy programmes, as compared with other treatments, in terms of women's quality of life for women who have experienced domestic violence

Ⓢ **Table 5.2** Sue's systematic review on witnessed resuscitation (qualitative review)

Problem statement	Little is known about the lived experiences of patients, family members and healthcare professionals regarding family presence during resuscitation and/or invasive procedures.
Review question	Family presence during resuscitation and/or invasive procedures: What is the lived experiences of patients, family members and healthcare professionals?
Aim	The aim of this systematic review is to evaluate the lived experience of patients, family members and healthcare professionals regarding family presence during resuscitation and/or invasive procedures.
Objectives	• Search for papers on the lived experiences of patients, family members and healthcare professionals.
	• Collect data on the lived experiences of patients, family members and healthcare professionals.
	• Compare the lived experiences of the different healthcare professionals.
	• Compare the findings of this systematic review with other systematic reviews.
	• Provide guidelines for nurses associated with family presence during resuscitation.
Title	A systematic literature review on family presence during resuscitation and/or invasive procedures: The lived experience of patients, family members and healthcare professionals.

When you have filled in all the details for your own systematic review question, read them again to make sure that for each section you are consistently using the same words and phrases throughout. It may be worth giving it to a colleague to read to see if they agree with you.

Box 5.3   Template for recording your problem statement, review question, aim, objectives and title for your systematic review

Problem statement

Review question

Aim

Objectives

Title

Specifying the inclusion and exclusion criteria for selecting primary research papers

Having stated your aims and objectives for your systematic review, the next step is to state your inclusion and exclusion criteria before you conduct the systematic review. This is important because of the following reasons:

- The inclusion criteria are the elements that the primary papers selected for the systematic review must meet to be included in the review, to ensure a quality systematic review.
- The exclusion criteria are essentially those factors that may impede or make the systematic review ineligible by not answering the systematic review question.

Following the PICOT and/or PEOT frameworks will help you focus on finding primary papers that enable you to answer your systematic review question. Examples of criteria can be found in Chapter 3, Step 4 (Criteria for considering studies for this review), page 67. Khan and Zamora (2022), similar to Torgerson (2003), suggest that a high-quality systematic review should have inclusion and exclusion criteria; these should be 'rigorously and transparently reported *a priori* (before you start the review)' (Torgerson 2003: 26). You may well ask: 'Why is this necessary?' The reason is so that your comprehensive search can target the primary research papers that will answer your systematic review question and exclude any irrelevant ones. The criteria need to be explicit and applied stringently (Kahn and Zamora 2022). The criteria need to be specifically stated for each element of the PICOT or PEOT acronym.

We would suggest that you write up your criteria in the following way. Start by describing the types of research study designs (T), including:

- the participants
- the intervention/s
- the comparative group/s (if any)
- the outcome measures.

Please note that whether you are writing a qualitative, quantitative or mixed-methods systematic review, the steps are the same, with the exception of qualitative reviews. This is because data extraction and presentation of results are conducted differently from quantitative reviews. Further information on these differences can be found in Chapters 7 and 8.

Specifying the inclusion and exclusion criteria for each component (PICOT or PEOT) of your systematic review question will now be discussed.

Specifying the types of studies to be included and excluded

When selecting your primary research papers, it is important to select papers that match the research design for your specific systematic review question. If you are evaluating the effectiveness of an intervention, the highest quality research designs will be randomized controlled trials (RCTs) or controlled clinical trials (CCTs). (Please refer to the hierarchy of evidence research design section in Chapter 2, in Box 2.8 and Figure 2.12, to go over the different research designs if you are still uncertain about this.) You could also use other research designs that do not include a control intervention, but these will be lower on the hierarchical scale of quality of evidence. In a Cochrane systematic review we conducted with an international team of colleagues, both RCTs and CCTs were included; we also included the prospective cohort study design because we knew that there were not many RCTs on this specific systematic review question (Romano et al. 2024).

In the case studies, Tamara and Mary will be seeking papers of a similar research design as they are looking at conducting – quantitative systematic reviews on the effectiveness of interventions. They have excluded case studies, because case studies are very low down on the quality-of-evidence scale. Despite this, however, if there are very few primary research papers available on your specific systematic review question, it may be worth considering the inclusion of case study designs. Essentially, if you end up finding no primary research papers on your systematic review question then your systematic review may end up being an 'empty' review.

In contrast, Sue will be evaluating people's lived experiences of witnessed resuscitation and will be conducting a qualitative systematic review. If you plan to conduct a qualitative systematic review, you will be searching for primary qualitative papers. The specific type of qualitative paper (i.e. phenomenological, ethnographic or grounded theory, among others) will depend on your specific qualitative review question. Tables 5.3, 5.4 and 5.5 illustrate how the inclusion and exclusion criteria for the three different case studies can be presented. These can be presented in tables or in narrative format as you prefer.

T **Table 5.3** Tamara's inclusion and exclusion criteria for her scoliosis review (quantitative intervention study)

Type of studies	Include	Exclude
Quantitative	RCTs	Commentaries
	CCTs	Review documents
	Cohort	Case studies
		Qualitative studies

M **Table 5.4** Mary's inclusion and exclusion criteria for her domestic violence review (quantitative intervention study)

Type of studies	Include	Exclude
Quantitative	RCTs	Commentaries
	CCTs	Review documents
	Cohort	Case studies
		Qualitative studies

S **Table 5.5** Sue's inclusion and exclusion criteria for her witnessed resuscitation review (qualitative study)

Type of studies	Include	Exclude
Qualitative	Phenomenological	Letters
	Grounded theory	Commentaries
	Descriptive	Reviews
	Ethnography	Discussion papers
		Quantitative studies

Specifying the types of participants to be included and excluded

T To explain this process let's begin by discussing Tamara's case study. Tamara plans to include only children and adolescents aged 10 years of age or older when diagnosed. She makes it clear that the primary research papers she needs to find will include only those related to adolescents or children. She is also specifying that the age limit for including children will be either until they stop growing (as measured by pelvis or wrist radiographs or both) or until they are 18 years old (she referred to the definition provided by the Scoliosis Research Society). Tamara also needs to be specific as to the types of patients she will be excluding. She has decided to exclude any patients where scoliosis was not the primary diagnosis, such as congenital, neurological, metabolic and post-traumatic. Tamara's population inclusion and exclusion criteria can be seen in Table 5.6.

T **Table 5.6** Tamara's inclusion and exclusion criteria for her population

Review	Inclusion criteria	Exclusion criteria
Clinical population and diagnosis	*(State who the population will be and provide an operational definition)* Patients with AIS (i.e. patients who develop a curve and rib hump when they are 10 years of age or older and for which there is no known cause)	*(Specify what types of diagnosis will be excluded)* Adults with idiopathic or degenerative scoliosis and adolescents with any type of secondary scoliosis (e.g. neurological, metabolic, post-traumatic)
Age	*(Provide the upper and lower age limits, with a rationale)* Aged 10–18 or until the end of bone growth and measured by an X-ray of the wrist or pelvis	Children under 10, adults over 18 years of age and adolescents whose bone growth has ended
Stage or severity of disease	*(In some clinical conditions it is important to know how long patients have had the disease, as the symptoms are likely to be more severe the longer the patients have had the disease)* All curve types and magnitudes	Curves >50 degrees
Other factors relevant to your population group	*(Include any factors that are important for the reader to know)* As defined by the British Scoliosis Society and Scoliosis Research Society	

S Let us now consider Sue's review on witnessed resuscitation. Sue plans to include adult patients over the age of 18 years up to the age of 60 years. She thinks that patients younger or older than this age range may have perceptions that are quite different. Sue needs to provide the operational definition again, which in her case is 'resuscitation or invasive procedures', as well as the setting, which will be 'within a tertiary setting (hospital)'. She must also specify the type of injury: 'after suffering cardiac arrest or substantial injury warranting a lifesaving intervention'.

Finally, as Sue will be looking into the perspectives of three different populations – that is, the patient, the family members and the healthcare professionals – she needs to specify who these will be. Family members will include spouse, partner, close friend, carer, parent, sibling, son and daughter. Healthcare professionals will include any named nurse, charge nurse, nurse practitioner or sister whose role is advocating for the patient and who is part of the resuscitation team or is involved with the patient and family in the capacity of delivering a 'duty of care'. Other healthcare professionals would include consultants, specialists, doctors, surgeons, physiotherapists, social workers or occupational therapists. Sue has decided to include the perspectives of all the different types of healthcare professionals.

As shown in Table 5.7, Sue plans to include three different population groups so that she can explore the experiences of all three groups and also to evaluate if there are differences in perceptions among them.

§ **Table 5.7** Sue's criteria for the three different population groups specified for her review on witnessed resuscitation

Review	Inclusion criteria	Exclusion criteria
Population 1 *Patient*	Adult patients >18 years undergoing cardiopulmonary resuscitation/invasive procedure	Children <18 years, patients undergoing chemotherapy, patients suffering from chronic illness or who have a DNAR (do not attempt resuscitation). Layperson, onlooker, hospital porter, ward clerk
Population 2 *Family members*	Spouse, partner, close friend, carer, parent, sibling, son, daughter	Bystanders, friends
Population 3 *Healthcare professionals*	Named nurse, charge nurse, nurse practitioner, sister, consultant, specialist, doctor, surgeon, physiotherapist, social worker, occupational therapist	Ward clerk, porters, housekeepers, priests

In Table 5.8 Mary records the population criteria for her domestic violence review.

In summary, when describing the inclusion and exclusion criteria for your population(s) in your systematic review, it is important that you clearly state who the population(s) will be and that you specify their diagnosis, the severity and duration of the disease, who will be included as well as any other relevant factors, as discussed above. Box 5.4 contains a template for you to use in recording your population criteria.

Ⓜ **Table 5.8** The population criteria for Mary's domestic violence review

Review	Inclusion criteria	Exclusion criteria
Population	Women	Men, children and teenagers
	Adults >18 years	Women in lesbian relationships and men in gay relationships
	Experiencing or have experienced domestic violence in the past	Women with disabilities, pregnant women

Box 5.4   Template for recording your own population criteria

Review	Inclusion criteria	Exclusion criteria
Clinical population	(State who the population will be and provide an operational definition)	
Diagnosis	(State and define the diagnosis)	
Age	(Provide the upper and lower age limits, with a rationale)	
Stage or severity of disease	(In some clinical conditions, it is important to know how long patients have had the disease, as the symptoms are likely to be more severe)	
Other factors relevant to your population group	(These can include any other factors that you think are important)	

Practice session 5.2

Use the template in Box 5.4 for writing down the population criteria for your own review.

Specifying the interventions (or exposure) to be included and excluded in your systematic review

You could start this section by first describing the interventions you plan to include in your review. Tamara's example is shown in Table 5.9.

T **Table 5.9** The criteria for Tamara's intervention and comparative groups

Intervention	Inclusion criteria	Exclusion criteria
Intervention	All types of rigid, semi-rigid and elastic braces, worn for a specific number of hours, for a specific number of years	Electrotherapy traction Exercise only
Comparative intervention	All possible control interventions and comparisons were included	None

M With regards to Mary's review on domestic violence, she provides a brief explanation of what is meant by 'community advocacy programmes' and then states which different types of programmes she will be including in her own systematic review. In this section it would also be useful for her to state clearly whether the papers she is planning to use will include *all* types of programmes or only those with particular characteristics, for example only those that are run by women who have themselves experienced domestic violence and not those run only by healthcare professionals. One way of presenting the inclusion and exclusion criteria for Mary's review on domestic violence is shown in Table 5.10.

M **Table 5.10** Mary's criteria for intervention and comparative intervention

Intervention	Inclusion criteria	Exclusion criteria
Intervention	Advocacy (conducted within or outside of health setting) Community programmes (need to include a clear definition of these)	Non-formal cognitive–behavioural therapy
Comparative intervention	Usually general practitioner (GP) treatment (usually this means no treatment for domestic violence)	Other interventions Alternative therapies

Another point to consider is whether or not you are planning to include interventions carried out all over the world or just those in the UK. Higgins et al. (2023) recommends finding *all* available studies from all over the world, but if your specific review question relates to treatment methods conducted only within the UK, it is best to explain this and provide a rationale. Sue's inclusion and exclusion criteria for her systematic review on witnessed resuscitation are shown in Table 5.11; her inclusion criteria are very comprehensive.

§ **Table 5.11** Sue's inclusion and exclusion criteria for her exposure criteria

	Inclusion criteria	Exclusion criteria
Exposure: Witnessed cardiopulmonary resuscitation after patient suffers a cardiac arrest OR Invasive procedures performed while undergoing resuscitation or as a lifesaving measure	Tertiary setting, such as hospital intensive care unit (ICU), paediatric intensive care unit (PICU), maternity departments, coronary care unit (CCU), high-dependency unit (HDU), A&E departments, patient's home, ambulance or community setting	Hospice setting Rehabilitation establishment

Specifying the comparative interventions to be included and excluded

The comparative intervention only needs to be specified if you are using the PICOT format, and not if you plan to use the PEOT format. If you have a comparative intervention, you need to state the inclusion and exclusion criteria for the comparative intervention(s) you will be including within your review, together with your rationale. The comparative interventions for the two quantitative case studies can be seen in Tables 5.9 and 5.10.

Specifying the outcomes to be included and excluded

By outcome measures we are usually referring to measurable outcomes or clinical changes in health (Khan et al. 2003; Khan and Zamora 2022). Examples of outcome measures include body structures and functions like pain and fatigue, functional abilities, activities, participation and QOL measures, as seen in Box 5.5.

Box 5.5   Examples of types of outcome measures

You will need to state what type of outcome measures will be included; examples are listed below. It is important to highlight what the units of measurement are, i.e. length in mm, weight in kg, height in cm:

- **Body structures and functions:** Weight (kg), pain, fatigue
- **Activities:** Functional abilities, dexterity
- **Participation:** Physical independence, QOL
- **Process measures:** Compliance, strength
- **Other:** Rates of domestic violence
- **If it is a qualitative review:** Experiences and perceptions of subjects

In Sue's example the outcomes she will be looking at are the experiences, views or perceptions of her three different population groups (Table 5.12).

Table 5.12 Sue's 'outcomes' criteria for considering studies in her review based on the PEOT structure

Outcomes	Inclusion criteria	Exclusion criteria
Psychological issues, experiences, perceptions, views, feelings	Experiences, perceptions, views from all members of the population groups towards resuscitation and invasive procedures	Physical effects: insomnia, tachycardia, guilt

Mary's outcomes for the domestic violence intervention and review question are provided in Table 5.13.

Table 5.13 Mary's 'outcomes' criteria for considering in her review based on the PICO structure

Outcomes	Inclusion criteria	Exclusion criteria
Quantitative	Validated quality-of-life (QOL) scales (need to specify which ones)	Qualitative experiences

Box 5.6 shows how Tamara could write out her own outcome measures. Note that the references used in the case extracts are for illustrative purposes only and are not included in the reference list at the end of this chapter.

Practical Tip

Note that it is not enough to state that you will be measuring 'quality of life'. You also need to add what standardized assessment tools or validated measuring instruments will be included. It is important to include scales that are known to be reliable and valid, as those that are not could bias your results.

T Box 5.6   Tamara's outcome measures

Progression of scoliosis as measured by:

- the Cobb angle in degrees (the Cobb angle was devised by a surgeon, John Cobb, and measures the curvature of the spine)
- number of patients who have progressed by more than five degrees Cobb.

QOL and disability as measured by:

- specific validated QOL questionnaires such as SRS-22 (Asher et al. 2003), SF-36 (Lai et al. 2006), and BSSK (Weiss and Werkmann 2007).

Back pain as measured by:

- validated visual analogue scales (visual analogue scales provide a simple technique for measuring subjective experience; see McCormack et al. 1988)
- use of medication
- adverse effects, as measured in the identified papers, which will be reported.

Useful resources associated with nursing outcomes

Oner, B., Zengul, F.D., Oner, N., Ivankova, N.V., Karadag, A. and Patrician, P.A. (2021) Nursing-sensitive indicators for nursing care: A systematic review (1997–2017). *Nurs Open* 8: 1005–1022.

Kidd, L. (2023) Measuring what matters in person centred care, Blog, *Evidence-Based Nursing*, 2 July 2023. Available at https://blogs.bmj.com/ebn/2023/07/02/measuring-what-matters-in-person-centred-care/ (accessed 18 October 2023).

Cribb, A. and Woodcock, T. (2022) Measuring with quality: The example of person-centred care. *J Health Serv Res Policy* 27 (2): 151–156.

Finally, we will discuss Fay's review on catheter-associated urinary tract infection (CAUTI). The protocol for Fay's literature review was shown in Chapter 3. In the section below we have included Fay's own introduction to this section of her dissertation, as it provides a good example.

Note: As Fay completed this systematic review a while ago, it is important to highlight that any guidelines/recommendations will be outdated or will have been changed. We suggest that you if want to access the information you look for new updated materials in this area. Fay's references within the examples provided in this text are purely for illustrative purposes and are thus not included in the reference list.

F Fay's case study on CAUTI

Fay is a fictitious name for a student nurse who studied Bachelor of Nursing Science a number of years ago, as previously mentioned on page 61. Fay undertook a systematic review and kindly gave permission for us to use her systematic review question and thesis, as discussed in Chapter 3 where we reproduced her protocol. We believe her work helps significantly to illustrate key aspects of the systematic review process. Although we acknowledge that her thesis requires updating (with regards to her references and other policy developments) we are also of the opinion that her work offers sound insights into undertaking a systematic review. She had encountered many patients with CAUTIs both during her placements in hospital and in her placements in the community and was a little confused by the recommendations in place for catheter insertion at the time. Her area of interest was UTIs. The aim of her review was to evaluate the existing guidelines (back in 2008) that promoted the practice of *not* using antiseptics at catheter insertion. So her research question was: 'In patients requiring urinary catheterization, is sterile catheter insertion more effective than non-sterile insertion at reducing the incidence of catheter-associated urinary tract infection (CAUTI)?'

The following is an extract from Fay's introduction to her chapter on specifying her inclusion and exclusion criteria:

> The criteria for the selection of studies to be included in a systematic review need to be defined ahead of the selection process in order to avoid selection bias (Khan et al. 2003, pg 29). The components of the structured question are used to generate a list of selection criteria. Using the PICOT framework facilitates the process. The study types or designs are identified after considering their likely suitability for answering the systematic review question and their level on the evidence hierarchy, while also bearing in mind the probable abundance or scarcity of the relevant studies. Torgerson (2003, pg 27–28) recommends a rapid scoping of the literature early in the planning stage to establish how plentiful relevant studies are. This also serves to identify existing reviews; however, Torgerson also warns that this could be a source of bias in the review.

Commentary on Fay's inclusion and exclusion criteria

For ease of use, the inclusion and exclusion criteria for Fay's case study have been copied into Table 5.14. Please note that the columns headed 'Inclusion' and 'Exclusion' contain what Fay wrote in her dissertation, while the column headed 'Commentary on Fay's criteria' contains our commentary.

Table 5.14 Student nurse Fay's inclusion and exclusion criteria for each component of PICOT

	Inclusion	Exclusion	Commentary on Fay's criteria
T	Comparative studies: RCTs; prospective CCTs; cohort studies with a control group; case study with a control group; any prospective studies with a control group	Single-group studies; cohort studies without a control; qualitative studies	The best study designs to answer review questions regarding the effectiveness of an intervention are comparative studies; these studies compare the effect of the intervention on an outcome in the study group with the same outcome in the control group (who are not exposed to the intervention being assessed). Such studies feature high on the hierarchy of evidence when allocation to the two groups is randomized and concealed (RCTs); bias is avoided since any confounding variables are equally distributed between the two groups (Craig and Smyth 2007: 89–92). However, following a rapid scope of the literature, it was evident that studies relevant to the review question were unlikely to be numerous; therefore it was deemed necessary that other designs (shown on the left) which are not considered as sound as RCTs also be included. In other words, Fay has included most quantitative study designs that were prospective and with a control group, even case studies, as otherwise she risked not finding enough studies for her review.
P	Male or female patients undergoing urinary catheterization performed by a healthcare worker Short-term/long-term indwelling or intermittent catheterization Setting: hospital, rehabilitation unit or nursing home	Intermittent self-catheterization, suprapubic catheterization, pre-existing UTI, urological surgery, patients on antibiotics	Both male and female patients were included, as Fay wanted to know the outcomes for both genders. She has also specified that this needed to be done by a health worker. Why do you think she is stating this? She is stating this so as to try and make her study as free from error as possible and make the group she is including as similar as possible. If the patient or a family member performed the procedure this may have introduced more bacteria than if it had been done by a healthcare worker. Patients who required and underwent urinary catheterization, whether indwelling (short term or long term) or intermittent, and which was performed by a healthcare worker were included in the review. However, patients who underwent intermittent self-catheterization were excluded, along with those having pre-existing UTIs, those who had undergone urological surgery and those who were on antibiotics.

(continued)

⊩ Table 5.14   Continued

I	Sterile urethral catheterization	The interventions under investigation were the sterile or aseptic catheter insertion technique and the specific steps involved in the process, namely hand washing, sterile gloves and gowns, antiseptic meatal cleansing and use of antiseptic lubricating gel.
C	• Non-sterile urethral catheterization • Hand washing is omitted or modified and/or • no sterile gloves are used and/or • no sterile gowns are used and/or • no antiseptic meatal cleansing and/or • lubricating gel used contains no antiseptic	Non-sterile or clean catheter insertion techniques were the comparisons or controls examined; these included insertion techniques or their component steps that did not use antiseptics or sterile equipment as used in the sterile technique. Also included were insertion techniques where one or more of the specific steps of the sterile approach were either omitted or modified and/or where any of the processes mentioned in the inclusion criteria for the comparative intervention, seen on the left, occurred.
O	CAUTI confirmed by significant bacteriuria or clinical symptoms or urethral colony counts	The rate of incidence of CAUTI was considered as the outcome measure. CAUTI was identified as established by the presence of its clinical symptoms and/or the presence of significant bacteriuria. Significant bacteriuria was defined as 100,000 CFU/ml and was considered to be more reliable at diagnosing CAUTI, since the latter may be asymptomatic. It was assumed that CAUTI which could safely be attributed directly to catheter insertion would occur within the first few days following insertion and hence urine samples showing significant bacteriuria within this period would be most reliable.
	Other forms of catheterization	
	Any other outcomes	

Practice session 5.3

For your own systematic review question, select the appropriate template (PICOT or PEOT) and write out the inclusion and exclusion criteria for all the PICOT (Box 5.7) or PEOT (Box 5.8) components below.

Box 5.7   PICOT template to use for your own inclusion and exclusion criteria

	Inclusion criteria	Exclusion criteria
Population		
Intervention		
Comparative groups		
Outcome		
Type of studies		

Box 5.8   PEOT template to use for your own inclusion and exclusion criteria

	Inclusion criteria	Exclusion criteria
Population		
Exposure		
Outcome		
Type of studies		

Key points

- A problem statement is a simple statement of 'what is.'
- The review question follows from the problem statement.
- The aim of a project is to solve the problem and answer the review question.
- The objectives are usually more specific than the aim.
- The objectives state what the researcher is going to do.
- Your aims and objectives need to be written clearly and concisely.
- Always make sure you can identify the PICOT or PEOT elements within your aims and objectives.
- When writing your objectives, think of what it is you will actually be doing.

- Ensure that your aims, objectives, research question and title are all saying the same thing. The best way of doing this is to use virtually the same words for all four.

- A high-quality systematic literature review should have inclusion and exclusion criteria that are reported before the review is conducted – that is, a priori.

- It is important that your search can target the papers that will answer your question and exclude any irrelevant ones.

- The inclusion and exclusion criteria for your review need to be explicit and applied stringently. They need to be articulated for each component of PICOT or PEOT.

Summary

This chapter discussed the meanings of and differences between a problem statement, a review question, aims and objectives. Methods of specifying the inclusion and exclusion criteria for the types of studies, the population(s), intervention, comparative intervention(s) or exposures, and outcome measures were discussed. Examples were provided for different quantitative and qualitative review questions. Templates were provided to help you write out your own problem statement, aims, objectives and inclusion and exclusion criteria.

Question and Answer (Q&A)

(Q) What are the pitfalls that may result from not having identified clear inclusion and exclusion criteria?

(A) Articulating clear inclusion and exclusion criteria enables you to identify, locate and choose the most relevant primary research papers to answer your systematic review question. Having unclear inclusion and exclusion criteria has the potential to impact the quality and outcomes of the final systematic review. Clear criteria also help to ensure that the process you use to select your papers for inclusion/exclusion within your own systematic review is always based on the same criteria. If the criteria are not clear, then you may find that you will select some papers based on the original inclusion criteria and then select other papers based on different, unwritten criteria. This type of selection could culminate in introducing bias into the process of selecting and including your papers. For instance, if you found a paper written by a famous professor in a very similar area but not strictly meeting all your inclusion criteria, then you may be tempted to include it in your systematic review.

References

Davies, A. (2019) Carrying out systematic literature reviews: An introduction. *British Journal of Nursing* 28 (15): 1008–1014.

Higgins, J.P.T., Thomas, J., Chandler, J. et al. (eds) (2023) *Cochrane Handbook for Systematic Reviews of Interventions*, version 6.4 (updated August 2023). Available at www.training.cochrane.org/handbook (accessed 18 October 2023).

Jenkins, S., Price, C.J. and Straker, L. (1998) *The Researching Therapist: A Practical Guide to Planning, Performing and Communicating Research*. Edinburgh: Churchill Livingstone.

Khan, K.S. and Zamora, J. (2022) *Systematic Reviews to Support Evidence-Based Medicine: How to Appraise, Conduct and Publish Reviews*, 3rd edn. London: Royal Society of Medicine Press.

Khan, K.S., Kunz, R., Kleijnen, J. and Antes, G. (2003) *Systematic Reviews to Support Evidence-Based Medicine: How to Review and Apply Findings of Healthcare Research*. London: Royal Society of Medicine Press.

Romano, M., Minozzi, S., Bettany-Saltikov, J. et al. (2024) Therapeutic exercises for idiopathic scoliosis in adolescents. *Cochrane Database of Systematic Reviews* 2: Art. CD007837. DOI: 10.1002/14651858.CD007837.pub3.

Torgerson, C. (2003) *Systematic Reviews*. London: Continuum.

6

Conducting a comprehensive and systematic literature search

Overview

- The importance of undertaking a comprehensive and systematic literature search
- The aims of undertaking a comprehensive and systematic literature search
- Key factors to consider when undertaking a comprehensive literature search
- Steps involved in converting your systematic review question into a comprehensive search strategy

The importance of undertaking a comprehensive and systematic literature search

When you conduct a systematic review, it is important that you try to retrieve all studies (or as many as possible) relating to the specific systematic review question that your systematic review is addressing. This means searching internationally (unless you are focusing on a specific country), as widely as possible from a whole range of sources. These include all the different websites and databases identified in Chapter 1, Box 1.2. Although you may eventually exclude some papers (if they do not meet all your inclusion criteria, as identified in Chapter 5) it is important that all the relevant studies are found and considered to ensure that your sample (all the studies you include) is as unbiased as possible. It is necessary to search a wide variety of databases and internet search engines as well as hand searching. This may involve online or manual page-by-page reviewing of the entire contents of a journal issue or an article to identify all eligible reports of published primary research. These may be located in abstracts, news columns, editorials, letters, other texts or other grey literature such as conference papers, symposiums quality reports, and so forth (Higgins et al. 2023).

The search strategy provides a platform for performing your overall search in a logical and accurate way. A thorough and complete search strategy is *imperative*, for the following reasons. The search strategy enables you to search widely and meticulously, as not all research is indexed in major databases and/or published in journals. Therefore, the information may not be easily retrievable. It is also worth noting that there may be long delays before papers are accepted for publication and published. Similarly, this could apply to publication gaps after conference presentations, which are common, because it takes authors a considerable amount of time to write up their findings, submit them, get them reviewed and then amend them as necessary. However, discovering a conference paper before the publication of the full paper could be important, as it may provide some, although maybe limited, information surrounding your topic and review question.

Practical Tip

Before starting your systematic literature search, we would suggest that you contact your local or university library to see if they offer a workshop or course or have any available information on how to help you undertake a literature search. We would encourage nursing and/or health and social care students to seek out their representative librarian for support with their search strategy. This is important to enable you to become familiar with searching for evidence on different health and social care databases, such as the Cumulative Index to Nursing and Allied Health Literature (CINAH) and the Allied and Contemporary Medicine Database (AMED). EBSCO (an acronym for Elton B. Stephens Company) is a highly accessed platform used by academic and government institutions because it contains numerous research databases, e-journals and academic resources. This could save you a great amount of time in the long term. Seeking out and accessing this type of support early on in your systematic review process will pay dividends in the longer term.

The aims of undertaking a comprehensive and systematic literature search

The aim of the systematic literature search, as outlined in Chapter 1, is to generate a comprehensive list of *primary* studies, both published and unpublished, that may be suitable for answering your proposed systematic review question. To be systematic and to minimize selection bias, the search must be comprehensive. 'Comprehensive' in this context is about ensuring and maintaining the validity and outcomes of your systematic review. This is dependent on the thoroughness and accuracy of your search strategy in generating all the relevant studies from the database searches. Conducting a comprehensive literature search helps to identify current knowledge relating to the relevant concepts and contexts about what is known and unknown in a particular field (Davies 2019).

A comprehensive search strategy, according to Higgins et al. (2023), underlies and enhances the quality of the systematic review, but the search can also impede the quality of your review if not undertaken correctly. Conducting a comprehensive review question and search strategy may be influenced by a number of critical factors, like some of those identified in the following subsections.

Key factors to consider when undertaking your comprehensive literature search

A number of key factors need to be considered when undertaking a systematic search for relevant articles, including the following:

- Reading reference lists will enable you to identify source ideas and concepts that highlight the design of studies. Similarly, looking at the contents pages of journals is a good way of identifying ideas and potential knowledge gaps.

- Hand searching may help to avoid possible bias in keyword search systems. Keyword search systems like MEDLINE, EMBASE and CINAHL help reviewers to identify published studies more easily. According to Rutgers University (2023) 'hand-searching is a manual process of screening pre-defined and pre-selected peer-reviewed biomedical [nursing] journals, conference proceedings and other publications for relevant materials that have been missed during the indexing process.' Manual searching is imperative for several reasons: it helps you to locate poorly or inaccurately indexed or unindexed articles and makes the perusal of journal content pages as well as whole journal contents easier, making the manual processes more efficient. It is important to remember that the advances in innovation and technology surrounding the accessibility and availability of databases and other associated information are not infallible. Our recommendation is to *always* liaise with and seek the support of librarians and IT specialists.

- Accessing grey literature, for example conference proceedings and PhD theses, will provide smaller and unpublished studies that may still be robust enough to provide valuable information.

- Getting in touch with authors of key articles may lead to them providing access to some of their important but unpublished work.

- Talking to colleagues about who the experts are in your area is another good way of identifying potential sources of work.

Review question

Ensuring that your search strategy is based on your systematic review question is *critical*. This is because your review question needs to include all the key elements of PICOT (population, intervention, comparative intervention, outcomes and types of studies), PEOT (population, exposure, outcomes and types of studies) or any other appropriate acronym. Your review question and associated search strategy impact *all aspects* and *steps* of your systematic review, ultimately impacting on the quality and outcomes of the findings and conclusions of your systematic review.

Publication and language bias

Problems with searching include publication and language bias. Publication bias means that positive results tend to be published more frequently in journals than negative results (Bruce et al. 2018). Language bias refers to the fact that positive results are more likely to be published in English. The seminal work by Egger et al. (1997) identified that researchers who obtained statistically significant results in randomized controlled trials (RCTs) were more likely to publish in an English-language journal. Whilst some researchers and students may find it easier to read research papers in their own language and try to avoid obtaining and reviewing papers published in other languages, where possible we would strongly recommend trying to work your way around this situation. It is important to seek out published articles in other languages, rather than choosing the biased option of not including potential papers because they are not written in your own language. This type of approach is not recommended, especially when the use of free translation services may be available online, for example Google Translate. Alternatively, you may be able to find a colleague or friend to translate a paper.

Publication and language bias may also relate to the geographical coverage of journals and databases. Some journals and databases tend to publish articles originating primarily from certain countries. Bruce et al. (2008) highlighted that the MEDLINE database included 10 million references to journal articles, of which more than half (62 per cent) originated from the USA alone. (Note that a second edition of the book by Bruce et al. was published in 2018.) On checking this statistic in late 2023 we found that this had risen to 30 million journal articles, of which only 34 per cent originated from the USA (NLM 2023). Perhaps this downward trend is due to the fact that other countries are now publishing more widely and in greater numbers.

Steps involved in converting your systematic review question into a comprehensive literature search strategy

There are a number of steps involved in converting the systematic review question into a search strategy. The first step is to refer back to the keywords that will form the basis of the search. According to Briscoe (2023) a 'systematic review is only as good as the search for studies on which it is based. A flawed search may fail to identify relevant studies and subsequently lead to erroneous conclusions.' To prevent this from happening it is important to review your question and to identify and use the appropriate keywords, which should be aligned and systematically follow your PICOT or PEOT.

It is possible to conduct searches using both index terms and free-text searching. Index terms include terms used by electronic databases, which may not precisely match the terms in your systematic review question, for example on the Medical Subject Headings (MeSH) database in MEDLINE. King's College London (2024) provides an easily accessible library guide focusing on how to undertake a comprehensive search strategy in a sequential way. Lahlafi's (2007) work continues to be highly relevant today. This is because to ensure that a search is comprehensive and both sensitive and specific, free-text searching, using what is known as 'natural language' or language we use daily, should be used in addition to or instead of index-term searching. The following section provides an overview of all the steps involved in conducting a comprehensive search for your systematic literature review in nursing practice. This includes a discussion of the process as a whole, illustrated by two of the case studies introduced in previous chapters.

Step 1: Write out the systematic review question and identify the component parts (keywords and so forth)

As mentioned in Chapter 2, the first step is to write out the systematic review question and identify the PICOT or PEOT components. Templates are provided for both the PICOT and PEOT types of questions below. Referring back to two of the case studies (Mary and Tamara), these can be written out as shown in Tables 6.1 and 6.2.

Ⓜ **Table 6.1** Key components of Mary's intervention research question on domestic violence, based on the PICOT structure

P	I	C	O	T
Women who have experienced domestic violence	Advocacy programmes	General prac- tice or routine treatment	Quantitative quality of life	RCTs, CCTs Cohort studies (measured by the SF-36 scale)

Ⓣ **Table 6.2** Key components of Tamara's intervention research question on adolescent idiopathic scoliosis, based on the PICOT structure

P	I	C	O	T
Patients with ado- lescent idiopathic scoliosis	How effective is spinal bracing ...	... as compared with other treat- ments ...	... at reducing spi- nal curvature, rib hump and psycho- logical problems?	RCTs CCTs Cohort studies

Practice session 6.1

Once you have read Mary's and Tamara's examples, use one of the empty templates below (Boxes 6.1 and 6.2) to write out the components of your own systematic review question based on the PICOT or the PEOT structure.

Box 6.1   PICOT template to use for your own review question

P	I	C	O	T

Box 6.2 PEOT template to use for your own review question			
P	E	O	T

Step 2: Identify and include synonyms

The second step is to identify any synonyms (words that mean the same thing) for all the component parts (P, I, C, O, T or P, E, O, T) of the systematic review question. For example, other terms for 'scoliosis' are 'curvature of the spine', or 'spinal deformity'. An easy way of finding similar words is by using the thesaurus function in your word processor (if available) or by consulting a good thesaurus. It is essential to understand that any search needs to be both sensitive and specific. Sensitivity (in this context) refers to a search that picks up all the research articles that are potentially relevant. Specificity refers to a search that selects only those research articles that are directly relevant to your specific topic. It is important to identify all the synonyms relating to the question and then to combine them using specific words called Boolean operators: these are words used in searches to combine different keywords or phrases. The most common operators are the following:

- OR: finds citations containing either of the specified keywords or phrases (sensitivity).
- AND: finds citations containing all of the specified keywords or phrases (specificity).
- NOT: excludes citations containing specified keywords or phrases.

Practice session 6.2   Writing your own synonyms
Use one of the empty templates (Boxes 6.3 and 6.4) to write out the synonyms associated with your own systematic review question, based on the PICOT or PEOT structure.

Box 6.3 PICOT template to use to indicate the synonyms related to your own review question				
P	I	C	O	T

Box 6.4 PEOT template to use to indicate the synonyms related to your own review question			
P	E	O	T

The various steps will be identified using the case studies of Mary and Tamara.

Mary's case study: Identifying synonyms and combining keywords

M Mary is researching domestic violence and needs to identify synonyms for all the PICOT components of her research question (Table 6.1). She is having difficulty think-ing of synonyms, so she decides to use a thesaurus. To help her in this task she uses a template (Table 6.3). This template has a column for each letter of PICOT (these can also be called strings) and a row for each different synonym.

Using this type of template enables Mary to combine all the related terms of her systematic review question to try to obtain as many relevant articles as possible. It also optimizes the sensitivity and specificity of her search. To explain this further, let us refer back to her systematic review question. If we start with the population column P, Mary first needs to find synonyms for 'women who have experienced domestic violence'. Synonyms for this could include 'wife abuse', 'partner abuse', 'battered women' and 'spouse abuse'. In Table 6.3, Mary first creates a list under the heading of patient/condition with each synonym in a new row. Mary continues by including synonyms for each component of the review question (ie PICOT or PEOT). In Table 6.4 Mary numbers the synonyms for each component of PICOT/PEOT from 1 to 9 (there happen to be nine in this case). Numbering your synonyms enables you to sequence your search strategy to follow a more coherent series of steps.

Try and help her combine her keywords. Remember to start by splitting your review questions into its component parts.

Ⓜ Table 6.3 Template used by Mary to identify the synonyms for her review question

Column terms combined with	Patient/condition AND	Intervention AND	Comparative intervention AND	Outcomes AND	Type of studies
OR	Domestic violence	Treatment	General practice	Quality of life (QOL)	Quantitative studies
OR	Women who have experienced domestic violence	Advocacy programmes	General practice/routine treatment	Quantitative QOL scale	RCTs
OR	Wife abuse	Group support	GP	QOL	CCT
OR	Partner abuse	Individual support	Routine treatment	Happiness	Cohort studies
OR	Battered women	Advocacy programmes	Doctor	Sorrow	Case studies
OR	Spouse abuse	Counselling	Physician	Depressed	
OR	Rape	Community	Surgery	Anxious	
OR	Sexual abuse	Therapy			

Ⓜ **Table 6.4** Mary's completed template showing the *final number* used to identify the keywords and synonyms

Column terms combined with	Patient/ condition AND	Intervention AND	Comparative intervention AND	Outcomes	Type of studies
OR	1 Domestic violence	11 Treatment	21 General practice	28 Women's quality of life	35 RCTs
OR	2 Wife abuse	12 Group support	22 GP	29 QOL	36 CCT
OR	3 Partner abuse	13 Individual support	23 Routine treatment	30 Happiness	37 Cohort studies
OR	4 Battered women	14 Advocacy programmes	24 Doctor	31 Sorrow	38 Case studies
OR	5 Spouse abuse	15 Counselling	25 Physician	32 Depressed	
OR	6 Rape	16 Community	26 Surgery	33 Anxious	
OR	7 Sexual abuse	17 Therapy			
OR	8 Coercion	18 Support			
OR	9 Murder	19 Advocacy			
	10 Combine 1–9 using 'OR'	20 Combine 11–19 using 'OR'	27 Combine 21–26 using 'OR'	34 combine 28–33 Using OR	39 Combine 35–38 using OR

The last step is to combine steps 10+20+27+34+39 together using the term 'AND'.

The numbers represent the order or the individual steps of how the words will be typed into the search database (for example EBSCO or CINAHL) and have been included to help you understand how this process is conducted. This is repeated for the intervention 'I' (steps 11–19), the comparative intervention 'C' (steps 21–26), the outcomes 'O' (steps 28–33) and, lastly, the types of studies 'T' (35–38). When all the words in each of the five columns have been combined with 'OR', all the synonyms for P, I, C O and T are combined using the Boolean term 'AND'. Do make sure that after the last synonym for each string you include an additional number to allow space for the combinations. The final part of the search strategy is to combine steps 10+20+27+34+39 together using the Boolean term 'AND'. The process sounds very complicated but once you have worked through the two examples below (Tables 6.5 and 6.6), it should become easier and clearer.

Practical Tip

To improve your knowledge and skills of the above, we would recommend that you practise this process using other examples. There is no substitute for practice in regard to this process. Remember the saying: 'Practice makes perfect'.

Step 3: Identify truncations and abbreviations

Once you have identified your synonyms, the third step is to identify any truncations or abbreviations. Truncation in this context means cutting something short. The symbol $ is a shortcut termed 'truncation' and identifies variations of a word. What this means is if Mary, for example, searched using the word 'therapy', the search would only look for the word 'therapy' and leave out anything like therapeutic, therapist, therapists, and so forth. In a number of databases, you may find that the truncation is indicated with a star * at the end of the word. Please make sure that you read all the relevant information specific to the database before you use it to ensure that you are using the correct truncation sign. Most libraries, especially university ones, have library guides for different databases, along with information on how to conduct your search effectively.

Practical Tip

If in doubt, consult with a librarian. Do not hesitate to talk to your librarian.

Mary was finding this part difficult, so she looked at other systematic reviews on a similar topic and also used a hard-copy thesaurus (these tend to be much more comprehensive than online ones) and a dictionary to help her to find synonyms or words of similar meaning. Going back to Mary's example, her truncations ($ dollar sign in bold) can be seen in Table 6.5. If you find this part quite hard, there is no need to worry. This step is not absolutely necessary, because you can also conduct the search using the key terms without any abbreviations: it will just take a bit longer. Sometimes, it is also necessary to identify abbreviations that are commonly used. For example, the intervention 'cognitive behavioural therapy' is frequently found as CBT in the literature. It is important at this stage to recognize that a number of words and phrases may be spelt slightly differently in other countries. For example, in American English behavior is spelt without the letter U.

Tamara's case study: Identifying synonyms

As with Mary's case study, Tamara begins by identifying the key components of her systematic review question (Table 6.2) and then starts identifying the synonyms for her keywords. Tamara's **P**opulation group are patients with adolescent idiopathic

Ⓜ **Table 6.5** An example of how Mary could identify truncations for her key terms

Column terms combined with	Patient/ condition AND	Intervention AND	Comparative intervention AND	Outcomes	Type of studies
OR	1 Domestic violence	11 Treatment	21 General practice	28 Women's quality of life	35 RCTs
OR	2 Wife abuse	12 Group support	22 GP	29 QOL	36 CCT
OR	3 Partner abuse	13 Individual support	23 Routine treatment	**30 Happ$**	37 Cohort studies
OR	4 Battered women	**14 Advocacy prog$**	**24 Doctor$**	31 Sorrow	38 Case studies
OR	5 Spouse abuse	**15 Counsel$**	**25 Physician$**	**32 Depress$**	
OR	6 Rape	**16 Com$**	**26 Surg$**	33 Anxious	
OR	7 Sexual abuse	**17 Ther$**			
OR	8 Coercion	18 Support			
OR	9 Murder	**19 Advoc$**			
	10 Combine 1–9 using 'OR'	20 Combine 11–19 using 'OR'	27 Combine 21–26 using 'OR'	34 Combine 28–33 Using OR	39 Combine 35–38 using OR

The last step is to combine steps 10+20+27+34 +39 together using the term 'AND'.

scoliosis (AIS). As is shown in Table 6.6, she writes this under the population heading (column) and numbers it (1). What other synonyms are there for AIS? She could use:

- (2) 'spinal deformity'
- (3) 'spinal curvature'
- (4) 'lateral curvature'
- (5) 'crooked spine'
- (6) 'rib hump'
- (7) 'poor posture'
- (8) combine 1-7 using OR.

Tamara now needs to combine all the synonyms using the Boolean operator 'OR' (see Table 6.6). This simply means that she is asking the search engine to search for any papers that have as a population group any of the synonyms listed. So, this will be step 8 and can be written as [combine 1–9 using 'OR']. In other words, she is trying to make

her search as sensitive as possible. The Boolean operator 'OR' finds citations containing any of the specified keywords, phrases or synonyms (sensitivity).

Tamara's next step is to repeat this process for the Intervention, Comparative
Interventions, Outcomes and Types of study columns on the template. The word
'brace' under the intervention heading will now be step 9, the word 'rigid brace' will
now be step 10, 'semi-rigid brace' step 11, 'soft brace' step 12 and 'spinal orthosis' step
13. Tamara cannot think of any more synonyms or find any more in the thesaurus, so
she now needs to let the search engine know that she would like to look for any of the
listed synonyms for the word 'brace'. Tamara will now write this as follows: step 16
combine [9–16 using 'OR'] and will write them in the intervention column below (Table
6.6, see page 147 for Tamara's full search strategy list).

Tamara continues doing this for the comparative intervention column, outcomes,
and types of study. The last step is for her to combine all the 'OR' combinations for each
column (10+20+27+34+39) using the Boolean operator 'AND', which will find citations
containing all of the specified keywords or phrases (specificity). To summarize, this
will enable Tamara to make her search as sensitive and specific as possible in order to
enable her to find as many relevant citations as possible to answer her review question.

T **Table 6.6** Template used by Tamara to start identifying keyword synonyms

Column terms combined with	Patient/condition AND	Intervention AND	Comparative intervention AND	Outcomes AND	* Type of study designs AND
OR	1 Patients with adolescent idio-pathic scoliosis (AIS)	9 Brace	16 Exercise	23 Reduces curvature	29
OR	2 Spinal deformity	10 semi-rigid brace	17 Scoliosis-specific exercise	24 Rib hump	30
OR	3 Spinal curvature	11 Soft brace	18 Physiotherapeutic scoliosis-specific exercise	25 Angle of trunk rotation	31
OR	4 Lateral curvature	12 Spinal orthosis	19 Schroth sco-liosis-specific exercises	26 Balance	32
OR	5 Crooked spine	13 Asymmetrical brace	20 SEAS (scientific exercise approach to scoliosis)	27 Quality of life	
OR	6 Rib hump	14 Symmetrical brace	21 FITS (functional independent ther-apy for scoliosis)		
OR	7 Poor posture				
	8 Combine1–7 using 'OR'	15 Combine 9–14 using 'OR'	22 Combine 16–21 using 'OR'	28 Combine 23–27 using 'OR'	

The last step is to combine steps 8+15+22+28+32 together using the term 'AND'.

*You will notice that we have left the final column study designs empty for you to complete. These could include, for example, RCTs),
controlled clinical trials (CCTs), cohort studies and case studies. What component has Tamara left out?

Practice session 6.2

Now that we have discussed two examples, turn to your systematic review question that you developed in Chapter 2. Identify the synonyms, truncations and combinations for your keywords using one of the templates provided. There are two templates: one for PICOT and one for PEOT, in Boxes 6.5 and 6.6 respectively.

Box 6.5   PICOT template to use for your own review question to identify synonyms and combine keywords

Column terms combined with	Patient/ condition AND	Intervention AND	Comparative intervention AND	Outcomes AND	Types of studies
OR					
OR					
OR					
OR					

Box 6.6   PEOT template to use for your own review question to identify synonyms and combine keywords

Column terms combined with	Patient/ condition AND	Exposure AND	Outcomes AND	Types of studies
OR				
OR				
OR				
OR				

Step 4: Develop a search strategy string

The fourth step is to develop a search strategy string (i.e. a list of words) to input into the different databases. Keywords and synonyms need to be 'translated' or 'tweaked' to develop a search strategy list.

Ⓜ The following list shows exactly which words Mary will be typing into a specific database (for example EBSCO, CINAHL or MEDLINE) to conduct her search and the order and combinations of how she will type them in. Following on from the templates above (Tables 6.4 and 6.5), Mary first types the words from numbers 1 to 9 individually into the database search engine. Once she has done this she will need to combine them using the word 'OR' (line 10). This is repeated for the remaining columns – intervention I (20), comparative intervention C (27), outcomes O (34) and types of studies T (40). Once she has done this, all the PICOT synonyms need to be combined using the term 'AND', which means she will need to combine the numbers 10, 20, 27, 34 and 39. Mary's sequence for doing this is shown below:

Population

1 Domestic violence
2 Wife abuse
3 Partner abuse
4 Battered women
5 Spouse abuse
6 Rape
7 Sexual abuse
8 Coercion
9 Murder
10 **1 OR 2 OR 3 OR 4 OR 6 OR 5 OR 7 OR 8 OR 9 (Mary has combined terms using 'OR')**

Intervention

11 Treatment
12 Group support
13 Individual support
14 Advocacy programme
15 Counselling
16 Community
17 Therapy
18 Support
19 Advocacy
20 **11 OR 12 OR 13 OR 14 OR 15 OR 16 OR 17 OR 18 OR 19 (Mary has combined terms using 'OR')**

Comparative Intervention

21 General practice
22 GP
23 Routine treatment
24 Doctor
25 Physician

    26 Surgery
27 21 OR 22 OR 23 OR 24 OR 25 OR 26 (Mary has combined terms using 'OR')

Outcomes

    28 Women's quality of life
    29 QOL
    30 Happiness
    31 Sorrow
    32 Depressed
    33 Anxious
34 28 OR 29 OR 30 OR 31 OR 32 OR 33

Types of study

    35 RCTs
    36 CCTs
    37 Cohort studies
    38 Case studies
    39 Quality of life
    40 35–39 using OR
41 10 AND 20 AND 27 AND 34 and 40 (Mary has combined the terms using 'AND').

It is preferable to apply limits at the final stage of the literature search. Limits can include restricting the search to English-language articles, human studies or research articles and possibly specifying a date range (you will need to provide a rationale for this; it shouldn't just be arbitrary). For example, if there had been a significant change in advocacy programmes since 1990, it would be wise to limit the search strategy to articles written after this date. Different limits are available in different databases. If limiting a search to English-language articles only, it is important to acknowledge that a language bias has been introduced into the search as you may have left out potentially important and relevant articles written in other languages.

Practical Tip

You may want to consider using online language translation services to help you check titles, abstracts and other article details written in a language that you do not understand.

Practice session 6.3

With your own review question in mind, use the template in Box 6.7 to translate all the keywords and synonyms into a search strategy list like the ones developed by Mary and Tamara.

T Tamara's strategy list example can be found below:

Population

1 Patients with adolescent idiopathic scoliosis
2 Spinal deformity
3 Spinal curvature
4 Lateral curvature
5 Crooked spine
6 Rib hump
7 Poor posture
8 Combine 1–7 using 'OR'

Intervention

9 Brace$
10 Rigid brace$
11 Semi-rigid brace$
12 Soft brace$
13 Spinal orthosis
14 Orthopaedic device$
15 Orthopaedic equipment
16 Combine 9–15 using 'OR'

Comparative intervention

17 Exercise$
18 PSSE$
19 SEA$
20 FITS$
21 Electrical stimulation
22 Orthopaedic devices
23 Orthopaedic equipment
24 Combine 17–23 using 'OR'

Outcomes

25 Spinal curvature$
26 Rib hump$
27 Posture$
28 Back shape
29 Self-esteem
30 Self-confidence
31 Quality of life
32 Pain
33 Combine 25–32 using 'OR'

Types of studies

34 RCTs
35 CCTs
36 Cohort studies

37   Case studies
38   Combine 34–37 USING OR
39   Combine 8 AND 16 AND 24 AND 33 AND 39

Box 6.7   Template to use for translating your review question keywords into a search strategy list

---

Step 5: Undertake a comprehensive search using all possible sources of information

Having completed your search strategy string, the fifth step is to undertake a comprehensive search, using databases and all other sources of information that are of the highest priority to enable you to answer your review question. Sources of information fall into several categories, including:

- online general databases
- specialist databases
- journal articles
- PhD theses
- grey literature

- subject gateways
- conference papers and proceedings
- dissertation abstracts
- contacting experts (clinical and non-clinical)
- books.

Below is a brief description of each type of information source, together with a URL where you can access it.

General databases

Online databases include general databases like CINAHL, MEDLINE and AMED. An excellent publication titled 'Finding studies for systematic reviews: a checklist for researchers' is available on the website of the University of York's Centre for Reviews and Dissemination (CRD), at https://www.crd.york.ac.uk/CRDWeb/GuideToSearching. asp. This website contains a comprehensive list of the various websites and other sources of information you may need to access when undertaking a comprehensive search and review of the literature. A number of useful online databases are listed in Box 6.8. We would also like to refer you back to Box 1.2 in Chapter 1.

Box 6.8   Websites for some online health databases

- **MEDLINE:** This is the main source for bibliographic coverage of biomedical litera-ture; it covers numerous journals and specialties and has been in existence from around 1960. Available at https://www.nlm.nih.gov/medline/index.html.
- **CINAHL:** The Cumulative Index to Nursing and Allied Health Literature is a com-prehensive and authoritative resource for the professional literature of nursing, allied health, biomedicine and healthcare. Available at https://www.ebsco.com/products/research-databases/cinahl-database.
- **PsycInfo:** The American Psychological Association's PsycInfo database records professional and academic literature in psychology and related disciplines, includ-ing medicine, psychiatry, nursing, sociology, pharmacology, physiology and lin-guistics. Available at https://www.apa.org/pubs/databases/psycinfo.
- **AMED:** The Allied and Complementary Medicine Database covers a selection of journals related to physiotherapy, occupational therapy, palliative care and complementary medicine. Available at https://www.ebsco.com/products/research-databases/allied-and-complementary-medicine-database-amed
- **ASSIA:** The Applied Social Sciences Index and Abstracts website provides a com-prehensive source of social science and health information. Available at [https://about.proquest.com/en/products-services/ASSIA-Applied-Social-Sciences-Index-and-Abstracts/ (accessed 6 December 2023).
- **REHABDATA:** The National Rehabilitation Information Center (NARIC) produces the REHABDATA database, providing information on physical, mental and psychiatric disabilities, independent living, vocational rehabilitation, special

---

Box 6.8   (continued)

education, employment and assistive technology. Available at https://www.naric. com/?q=en/home (accessed 6 December 2023).

- **EBMR:** Evidence-Based Medicine Reviews is available at https://tools.ovid.com/ ebmr/lsmuni/ (accessed 6 December 2023).
- **CDSR:** You can access all issues in the Cochrane Database Of Systematic Reviews at https://www.cochranelibrary.com/cdsr/table-of-contents (accessed 6 December 2023).
- **DARE:** The Database of Abstracts of Reviews of Effectiveness, of the CRD of the University of York, can be accessed at https://www.crd.york.ac.uk/crdweb/ ShowRecord.asp?ID=32004000332 (accessed 6 December 2023).
- **ACP Journal Club:** The journal club of the American College of Physicians can be found at https://www.acponline.org/clinical-information/journals-publications/ acp-journal-club (accessed 6 December 2023).
- **CCTR:** The Cochrane Central Register of Controlled Trials is available at https:// www.cochranelibrary.com/central/about-central (accessed 6 December 2023).

Specialist databases

There are many online specialist databases covering particular medical specialties. For example, the National Cancer Institute website can be found at https://www. cancer.gov/.

Journal articles

Most of the searches you undertake on the databases identified above will direct you to primary research papers published in journals. We would suggest that journals are often regarded as primary sources containing the most up-to-date peer-reviewed information in all aspects of nursing. They may contain a mixture of primary and secondary research papers, including systematic reviews. They are a great resource in supporting you to undertake your systematic review that may be aligned to the professional nurse cycle, as detailed in Chapter 1 (see Figure 1.4 and Table 1.2).

Grey literature

Grey literature or non-journal literature refers to any unpublished sources of evidence. Most of the searches above focus on journal literature, but there are high rates of non-published research papers, and many PhD theses are not published; it is therefore essential to search the grey literature.

Grey literature refers to published abstracts, conference proceedings, policy documents, newsletters and other unpublished written material associated with your systematic review topic. OpenGrey, a system for information on grey literature, is an open-access website containing approximately 700,000 bibliographical references of grey literature (papers) produced in Europe. OpenGrey covers science, technology, biomedical science, economics, social science and humanities. OpenGrey is available at www.opengrey.eu/.

Subject gateways

Subject gateways provide access to reliable and up-to-date web resources for all subjects which have been carefully chosen and quality checked by experts in the fields. Subject gateways are also called subject guides, subject directories and subject portals. They allow you to browse subject topic lists of good quality and subject resources. Some of the more important nursing- and general-health-related subject gateways are listed in Box 6.9.

Box 6.9   Websites for some nursing- and general-health-related subject gateways

- **Nursing Portal (NP):** This is a gateway to the world of nursing. Available at www.nursing-portal.com (accessed 6 December 2023).
- **National Health Service (NHS) Knowledge and Library Hub (NHSKLH):** Available at https://library.nhs.uk/knowledgehub (accessed 6 December 2023).
- **Search Medica (SM):** This is an open-access medical search engine. Available at https://www.searchenginelinks.co.uk/search-medica-s553.html (accessed 6 December 2023).
- **Social Policy and Practice (SPaP):** This is an online database for evidence in health and social care. Available at http://www.spandp.net/ (accessed 6 December 2023).
- **Mentalhelp.net:** This website promotes mental health and wellness. Available at www.mentalhelp.net (accessed 6 December 2023).
- **Google Scholar and Google:** Two of the best-known general-purpose search engines, available at www.google.co.uk and scholar.google.co.uk (accessed 6 December 2023).

Conference papers and proceedings

The International Scientific Indexing (ISI) server provides indexing of major international journals and proceedings and access to quality-controlled open-access science and technology journals. The website contains details of approximately 10,000 conferences per year. The website is hosted by the University of Southern California, at https://isindexing.com/isi/ (accessed 6 December 2023).

Dissertation abstracts

The majority of university students undertake an extended research study or project resulting in a dissertation and/or thesis. The following website provides access to the abstracts of some dissertations which you may find useful: http://www.proquest.com/products-services/dissertations/ (accessed 6 December 2023).

Contacting experts (clinical and non-clinical)

The easiest way to contact experts and clinical and non-clinical specialists in your field of study is to Google their name to find a research paper that they have written. Most papers today include the contact details and corresponding email addresses for the lead author. Access to specific information may be limited online; you may have to approach the authors for permission to access or use their research work. Researchgate, an online repository for researchers and scholars, is also a useful database for finding specific researchers in a field. It is available at https://www.researchgate.net/ (accessed 6 December 2023).

Books

Books are useful secondary sources for identifying 'stable' types of information. They are a fantastic resource to aid you in the development of your introduction or background section of your systematic review. It is worth noting that some information in books may be dated, given the time involved from the writing of the manuscript to the final publication of the book. From our own experiences we know that a year or two years may go by from the time a manuscript is submitted to its final publication.

So, what are some of the challenges you might encounter when developing your search strategy?

On developing your outline strategy, we would recommend that you book an appointment with your librarian or information specialist if they are available. We have found this approach can potentially save you time, improve your overall strategy and outcomes and confirm that you are on the right track. For example, you may be doing everything right but still find no studies. In this case you could try a number of different things. You could leave the column containing the synonyms for the types of studies out of your search and redo your search. You may find that you will get more results. Similarly, you could try searching each string on its own first. This may give you an idea of how many references are available for each string. If when combining your terms you find that there are thousands of results, you may need to reconsider your search terms and/or add limits to the search. Again, if you have problems at this stage we recommend that you go and see a librarian or colleague with expertise in this area to support you.

Step 6: Save your searches

The final step is to record and save any searches as well as the results of the searches in an electronic format, so that all the necessary information is available and easily accessible when it comes to writing up your completed systematic review. The search strategy, including the database, the title of the article, the abstract, the host (for example OVID or EBSCO) and the date should be logged (see example in Box 6.10). As much detail as possible should be recorded, to enable a colleague or researchers to replicate your systematic review processes if required. Saving your valid search strategy is essential, especially if you need to cross-check or redo your search again at a later date. A discussion of the hits obtained and the selection process used to identify articles for closer scrutiny will provide an effective audit trail. Having an audit trail is imperative if someone wants to replicate your review.

Box 6.10   Example template of how you could document your first search

Database	Dates covered	Date searched	Hits	Full record/titles and abstracts	Notes
MEDLINE (EBSCO host)	1990–2012	20 March 2023	23	(Titles of the articles could be included here)	(You may want to give your search strategy a name, for example 'Medline1', just in case you need to run the search again sometime in the future)

Below is one way you could write up the databases you have searched:

- CINAHL (1982 to 12/2023)
- MEDLINE (1996 to 12/2023)
- British Nursing Index (BNI) (1994 to 12/2023)
- AMED (1986 to 12/2023)
- Proquest (1990 to 12/2023)
- PsycInfo (2000 to 12/2023)
- Scopus (1990 to 12/2023)
- EMBASE (1988 to 12/2023)
- Science Direct (1990 to 12/2023)
- PubMed (1996 to 12/2023)

Use Box 6.11 as a template for documenting your own search strategy for your systematic review.

Box 6.11   Template to use for documenting your search strategy

Database	Dates covered	Date searched	Hits	Full record/titles and abstracts	Notes

✐ Key points

- The aim of developing a robust systematic search from your review question is to generate a comprehensive list of primary studies, both published and unpublished, which may be suitable for answering the proposed review question.
- Try to retrieve all studies (or as many as possible) pertaining to addressing your specific review question, through searching as widely as possible in a range of sources and databases.
- It is necessary to search a wide variety of databases and internet search engines as well as undertaking hand searches and reviewing the grey literature.
- Problems with searching include publication and language bias.
- Publication bias means that positive results tend to be published more frequently than negative results in journals.
- Language bias refers to the fact that positive results are more likely to be published in English.
- Bias may also relate to the geographical coverage of journals and databases.
- Key activities include reading reference lists, hand searching, accessing grey literature and getting in touch with authors of key articles.
- There are six steps involved in converting the review question into a comprehensive search strategy.
  - o   Step 1 is to write out the systematic review question and identify the PICOT (population, intervention, comparative intervention, outcomes,

types of study) or PEOT (population, exposure, outcomes, types of study), or other associated component parts of your applied acronym.

o Step 2 is to identify any synonyms (words that mean the same thing) for all the component parts (P, I, C, O, T or P, E, O, T) of the review question.

o Step 3 is to identify truncations and abbreviations.

o Step 4 is to develop a search strategy string (list of words) to input into the different databases.

o Step 5 is to undertake your comprehensive search using all sources of information.

o Step 6 is to save your search strategy.

- Finally, seek the help and support of a librarian or information specialist if you are experiencing challenges at any stage.

Summary

This chapter has presented and discussed the importance, the rationale and the aims of undertaking a complete systematic search. The chapter described the key factors, based on the acronyms PICOT and PEOT, to be considered when undertaking your wide-reaching search. The six steps involved in converting your review question into a comprehensive search strategy were described in detail.

Question and Answer (Q&A)

(Q) Is there any support available to help me with searching for the evidence?

(A) There are useful and inexpensive ways available to help support you with searching the evidence:

- See if there are any literature searching sessions offered at your university, local hospital and/or university library.

- Contact a librarian or an information scientist for a one-to-one tutorial.

- Contact someone who has undertaken a systematic review within your place of work or study and ask them if they could provide any advice, guidance and support.

References

Briscoe, S. (2023) Errors to avoid when searching for studies for systematic reviews: A guide for nurse researchers. *International Journal of Older People Nursing* 18 (3): e12533.

Bruce, N., Pope, D. and Stanistreet, D. (2008) *Quantitative Methods for Health Research: A Practical Interactive Guide to Epidemiology and Statistics*. London: Wiley.

Bruce, N., Pope, D. and Stanistreet, D. (2018) *Quantitative Methods for Health Research: A Practical Interactive Guide to Epidemiology and Statistics*, 2nd edn. London: John Wiley and Sons.

Davies, A. (2019) Carrying out a systematic literature reviews: An introduction. *British Journal of Nursing* 8:28 (15): 1008–1014.

Egger, M., Zellweger-Zähner, T., Schneider, M., Junker, C., Lengeler, G. and Antes, G. (1997) Language bias in randomized controlled trials published in English and German. *The Lancet* 350 (9074): 326–329.

Higgins, J.P.T., Thomas, J., Chandler, J. et al. (eds) (2023) *Cochrane Handbook for Systematic Reviews of Interventions*, version 6.4 (updated August 2023). Available at www.training.cochrane.org/handbook (accessed 24 November 2023).

King's College London (2024) Searching for systematic reviews: Drawing up your search strategy. Updated 2 April 2024. Available at https://libguides.kcl.ac.uk/systematicreview/searchstrat (accessed 24 November 2023).

Lahlafi, A. (2007) Conducting a literature review: How to carry out bibliographical database searches. *British Journal of Cardiac Nursing* 2 (12): 566–569.

NLM (National Library of Medicine) (2023) MEDLINE® citation counts by year of publication (as of January 2023). Available at https://www.nlm.nih.gov/bsd/medline_cit_counts_yr_pub.html (accessed 24 November 2023).

Rutgers University (2023) Systematic reviews in the health sciences: What is hand searching? Available at https://libguides.rutgers.edu/c.php?g=337288&p=2269575 (accessed 24 November 2023).

7

Working with your primary papers: Stage 1 – Selecting the studies to include in your own systematic review

Overview

- Methods of the systematic review
- Selecting the appropriate papers to answer your systematic review question
- Templates to select the papers for your own systematic literature review

Methods of the systematic review

The methods section of the systematic review comprises three discrete stages, detailed in Figure 7.1. Chapters 7 to 9 describe these three stages. This chapter details Stage 1, selecting the studies to include in your systematic review, covering two steps: *Step 1* is selecting the papers from your search results by reading the titles and abstracts only and *Step 2* involves selecting the papers based on reading the full paper (Figure 7.2).

Stage 1	Selecting your papers	Step 1	Step 2
		(Based on titles and abstracts)	(Based on reading full papers)
Stage 2	Appraising your papers using a specific framework such as Caldwell et al., Critical Appraisal Skills Programme (CASP), McMasters		
Stage 3	Extracting data from your paper		

Figure 7.1 The three stages and steps of working with your primary papers.

Selecting the appropriate papers to answer your systematic review question

Once you have specified your inclusion and exclusion criteria, you can proceed to undertake your search to identify all the relevant primary studies. The next step is to select the primary research studies that meet all your predetermined selection criteria. The actual process of how you select the studies to include in your systematic review needs to be described in sufficient methodological detail. The latter ensures the following:

- It provides an auditable and transparent process, therefore enabling the steps to be easily replicated.
- It confirms the appropriateness of the methods used, which can therefore be more easily evaluated and duplicated.
- It provides a robust mechanism to filter out any irrelevant or duplicated articles.

Before you start
A standardized form needs to be made for *all* steps
This is important to standardize assessments between one paper and another
(i.e. improves inter- and intra-rater reliability)

Stage 1 – Step 1

At this point you have a large collection of abstracts, articles and papers from your search
1st Step – this selection is based on titles and abstracts ONLY considering the criteria of:

- type of study
- participants
- intervention
- comparative group
- outcome measures

using the standardized inclusion criteria *form*. Remember PICOT!
First selection can result in exclusion, inclusion or no decision on the title and abstract

Stage 1 – Step 2

This step is the same as for Step 1 but using the full papers. Second selection can result only in inclusion or exclusion of the full papers.

Figure 7.2 Flow diagram depicting the selection process.

As shown in Figures 7.1 and 7.2, the process of selecting studies for inclusion or exclusion in the review consists of two phases. The first phase involves sifting through the titles and abstracts of all the articles retrieved from the search, screening them systematically and selecting those that meet the predetermined inclusion criteria.

The second phase involves reading the full text of each identified article. For both phases it is useful to make an appropriate *research paper selection form* to help you standardize the way you select the articles that meet your predetermined criteria. This helps to make sure that you are always selecting the papers in the same way (i.e. it standardizes the process) and it also helps to improve the validity or truthfulness of the results.

Practical Tip

Developing a good study selection review template from the outset will enhance the quality and outcome of the review and make the process much simpler.

To explain how to make the paper selection form, let's look at examples from the three case studies used throughout this book – on domestic violence (Mary), adolescent idiopathic scoliosis (AIS) (Tamara) and witnessed resuscitation (Sue). Chapter 5 described how to specify your inclusion and exclusion criteria. In essence, to make your paper selection form all you need to do is copy the inclusion criteria and then turn these criteria into questions. Lets have a look at the case studies again:

Ⓜ In Mary's case study, she starts by finding the electronic copy of her inclusion and exclusion criteria (see, in Chapter 5, Tables 5.8, 5.10 and 5.13) and copies the first two columns: the columns stating the PICOT components and the inclusion criteria column. Mary then turns all her original listed inclusion criteria statements, as seen in Table 7.1, into questions (usually this can be as simple as adding a question mark), as can be seen in Table 7.2. Mary has added another row to the bottom of her table to record the action she will take, with the rationale. Mary has also added an additional column to the right side of the table (the decision column). This is to enable her to write whether or not the specific title and abstract meet the criteria (see Table 7.2). Mary's answers can be only one out of a possible three:

1   Yes, the paper meets these criteria (denoted by Y).
2   No, the paper does not meet these criteria (denoted by N).
3   Undecided as to whether this paper meets the inclusion criteria or not (denoted by U).

If Mary is undecided, she will need to read the whole paper as well as ask a colleague or a supervisor for their opinion.

Practical Tip

It is important to test your paper selection form on a couple of articles to make sure that it is fit for purpose (this is similar to conducting a pilot study when doing primary research).

Ⓜ **Table 7.1** Mary's original inclusion and exclusion criteria

PICOT components	Inclusion criteria	Exclusion criteria
Population	Women Adults >18 Experiencing or have experienced domestic violence in the past	Men, children and teenagers Women in lesbian relationships Women with disabilities Pregnant women
Intervention	Advocacy (conducted within or outside of health setting) Community programmes (need to include a clear definition of these)	Not formal cognitive-behavioural therapy
Comparative intervention	Usually (GP) treatment (usually this means no treatment for domestic violence)	Other interventions Alternative therapies
Outcomes Quantitative	Validated quality-of-life (QOL) scales (need to specify which ones)	Experiences only of domestic violence or of children only

Ⓜ **Table 7.2** An example of how Mary could write her study selection form

Paper number:	Title	Author
PICOT components	Inclusion criteria	Decision: Yes (Y), No (N), Undecided (U)
Population	Women? Adults >18? Experiencing or have experienced domestic violence in the past?	
Intervention	Advocacy (conducted within or outside of health setting)? Community programmes?	
Comparative intervention	Usually (GP) treatment (usually this means no treatment for domestic violence)?	
Outcomes	QOL?	
Action (with rationale)	Include (read full article), exclude or undecided	

Although it is perfectly possible to select your papers without using a template, it is important to remember that making or developing a screening template will strengthen the validity (truthfulness) of your results. You could ask a friend or colleague to review the papers independently to see if you both obtain the same results

(Khan and Zamora 2022; Higgins et al. 2023). If, however, you cannot find anyone to assist you, you should acknowledge this and state that because of this the validity of the results or selection of papers may have been decreased.

For Sue's case study on witness resuscitation, please refer back to the case study on Sue's review in Chapter 5.

§ Sue chose a slightly different format for her selection form (Table 7.3). Rather than making a template for one paper at a time, Mary decides to make a template to screen multiple papers at a time. She therefore uses one form to select a number of studies. Although she will use less paper, this format does have a few limitations. These are as follows:

- The amount of detail that she can include on her form is limited.
- She will need to add a key to the bottom of the form, to clarify which specific paper each number on the top row of the form represents.
- It may be difficult for her to write any specific queries that may arise from assessing each of her criteria for all her papers.

§ **Table 7.3** Sue's first selection of papers, based on title and abstract only

Paper and abstract number:	1	2	3	4	5	6	7	8	9	10	11
Population											
Adult patients	Y	N	?								
Age >18											
OR											
Family members OR	Y	Y	Y								
Healthcare professionals	Y	Y	Y								
Exposure											
Witnessed cardiopulmonary resuscitation or invasive procedures	Y	Y	?								
Outcomes											
Patient's experience of exposure	Y	Y	Y								
Family members' experience of exposure	Y	Y	Y								
Healthcare professionals' experience of exposure	Y	Y	Y								
Type of study											
Qualitative research	Y	N	Y								
***Action (decision)**	Y	N	U								

*Action – Rationale: Y = Yes: fits criteria; N = No: does not fit criteria; U = Unsure: read full paper.

After Sue has looked at three titles and abstracts, she fills in the first three columns on her selection form that represent these three papers (Table 7.3):

- In column 1 all the criteria have been met and Sue's overall decision (the action at the bottom) is to *include the paper.*
- In column 2 the action is *to exclude the paper* as two of the criteria have not been met.
- In column 3 there are two question marks, which means that Sue is undecided and needs to read the full paper and repeat the process. If she is still undecided after reading the full paper, she will need to consult with a colleague or supervisor to review the paper.

In summary, the first phase can result in including an article, rejecting it or being undecided and seeking a second opinion.

Once Sue has finished the first stage of the selection process, she will have a pile of abstracts of the following:

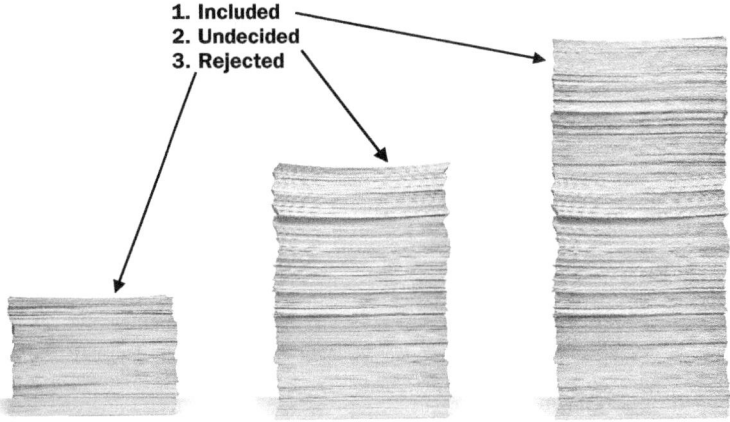

1. Included
2. Undecided
3. Rejected

The two piles of paper categorized as 'Included' and 'Undecided' must now be examined more closely for the second step of stage 1. This means obtaining full copies of the papers, reading them and making a decision regarding whether they meet *all the inclusion criteria* that have been pre-set (Higgins et al. 2023).

Ⴒ Tamara's paper selection form for her systematic review of adolescent patients with idiopathic scoliosis is shown in Table 7.4. Note that the references used in the case extracts are for illustrative purposes only and are not included in the reference list at the end of this chapter.

T **Table 7.4** Tamara's selection criteria for her primary papers

Bibliographic details of paper	Inclusion criteria	Decision: Yes, No, Undecided
Clinical population/ diagnosis	Patients with AIS?	
Age	Ages 10–18? Or until the end of bone growth? Measured by an X-ray of the wrist or pelvis?	
Intervention	Rigid brace? Semi-rigid brace? Elastic brace? Worn for how many hours per day? How many days per week? How many years?	
Comparative intervention	Exercise? Electrical stimulation? Surgery?	
Outcomes	Progression of scoliosis as measured by: • Cobb angle in degrees? • number of patients who have progressed by more than five degrees Cobb? QOL and disability as measured by? Specific validated QOL questionnaires such as: • SRS-22 (Asher et al. 2003)? • SF-36 (Lai et al. 2006)? • BSSK (Weiss et al. 2007)? Back pain as measured by: • validated visual analogue scales? • use of medication? • adverse effects?	
Type of studies	Randomized controlled trial (RCT)? Controlled clinical trial (CCT)? Cohort? Quasi-experimental?	
Action (with rationale)	**Include (read full article), exclude or undecided**	

Practice session 7.1

At this point you will probably have saved a number of papers from your searches and printed them out. Based on your own review question, use the appropriate template – for either the PICOT (Box 7.1) or PEOT (Box 7.2) format – to decide which of your primary research papers should be included, which will be excluded and which you are still undecided about (check these with a colleague to review independently). Once you have done this, you can go on to the next part of the study, which is reading the full papers and repeat the process of selection.

Box 7.1   PICOT template to use for your own selection of papers

Bibliographic details of paper *(Fill in the details of the paper you are evaluating here)*

	Inclusion criteria	Yes	No	Undecided
Participants	*(This is where you write down the criteria for your population details, diagnosis, age etc.)*			
Intervention	*(Here you write down the specific criteria for your intervention)*			
Comparative intervention	*(Same as above, but for comparative group)*			
Outcome	*(Write down the specific outcomes you are looking for)*			
Type of study designs	*(Write down the specific research designs you will be including)*			

(continued)

Box 7.1   Continued

Bibliographic details of paper *(Fill in the details of the paper you are evaluating here)*

	Inclusion criteria	Yes	No	Undecided
Action (with rationale)	*(The action will be yes, no or undecided for the first phase and yes or no only for the second phase)*			

Box 7.2   PEOT template to use for your own selection of papers

Bibliographic details of paper

Abstract number	1	2	3	4	5	6	7
Population (*Insert your own criteria in this column*)							
Exposure							
Outcomes							
Type of studies							
*Action							

*Action – Rationale: Y = Yes: fits criteria; N = No: does not fit criteria; U = Undecided, read full paper.

🔑 Key points

- There are three main stages to working with your primary research papers. The first stage involves selecting your articles, which is done in two steps.
- In Step 1, you develop an appropriate primary research paper selection template. This will aid you in standardizing the way you select the articles by reviewing the titles and abstracts, making your results more reliable and valid.
- Step 2 requires you to apply the above template for selecting your full primary articles. This involves sifting through the full primary studies retrieved from the search, screening them systematically and selecting those that meet the predetermined inclusion criteria.

Summary

This chapter focused on the first of three main stages that are involved in working with your primary research papers. The first stage includes ways of selecting appropriate papers to answer your review question. This step is conducted in two parts: first, selecting your papers based on the title and abstract according to your predetermined criteria and screening template, and secondly, reviewing the full papers. Developing and using the templates provided in this chapter will enhance this aspect of your systematic review.

Question and Answer (Q&A)

(Q) Are there any useful resources to aid in the selection of articles for a systematic review?

(A) There are several useful resources available to aid you in undertaking a quality systematic review of your articles. For example, the Joanna Briggs Institute and University of York's Centre for Reviews and Dissemination (CRD) both offer online resources and manuals highlighting the systematic review process.

References

Higgins, J.P.T., Thomas, J., Chandler, J. et al. (eds) (2023) *Cochrane Handbook for Systematic Reviews of Interventions*, version 6.4 (updated August 2023). Available at www.training. cochrane.org/handbook (accessed 24 November 2023).

Khan, K.S. and Zamora, J. (2022) *Systematic Reviews to Support Evidence-Based Medicine: How to Appraise, Conduct and Publish Reviews*, 3rd edn. London: Royal Society of Medicine Press.

8

Working with your primary papers: Stage 2 – Appraising the methodological quality of your included primary papers

Overview

- Appraising the methodological quality of the primary research papers that you have selected
- Worked example using the Caldwell framework to critique a nursing paper
- Actions during and following the completion of your critique

Appraising the methodological quality of the primary research papers that you have selected

As explained in Chapter 7, the methods-of-review section of your systematic review should cover the three separate stages detailed in Box 8.1. This chapter details Stage 2, focusing on how to identify and critique the methodological quality of your included primary research papers.

Box 8.1 Methods of the review

In this section you need to give details of the following three separate stages.

Stage 1: Description of the process of selecting the papers for inclusion in the systematic review. This stage has two steps. (See Chapter 7.)

Stage 2: Description of the process through which the methodological quality of the articles will be assessed.

Stage 3: Description of the process for the proposed data extraction strategy (see Chapter 9).

In the context of systematic reviews, quality refers to the methodological quality of the quantitative, qualitative or mixed-methods research papers that you have decided to include in your systematic review. Appraising 'study quality' is a phrase often used interchangeably with assessing the internal validity (quantitative) or trustworthiness (qualitative), which is the extent to which a research paper demonstrates its quality and freedom from methodological biases (Buccheri and Sharifi 2017) or the degree to which the results of a study are likely to approximate the 'truth' (Higgins et al. 2023).

With regards to quantitative studies, it is about establishing the internal and external validity of the research paper. Jadad (1998) suggested that the following points may be relevant when assessing the quality of the included quantitative papers; for example, when focusing on randomized controlled trials (RCTs) you may wish to consider the following:

- Relevance of the research question to the context of care – that is, clinical patients, practice area, speciality and wider nursing profession
- **Internal validity**, which is associated with the degree to which the RCT design, conduct, analysis and presentation have minimized or avoided bias
- **External validity**, which focuses on the extent to which findings from the RCT may be generalizable to inform other studies, practice and policy
- Appropriateness of the data analysis and presentation
- Ethical implications of the intervention of the research papers being evaluated. This refers to the ethical systems and processes in the included papers within the review; for example, was the research ethical approval and was informed consent obtained?

For more information on the above, see Texas A&M University (2024).

The criteria for appraising qualitative articles are different. Qualitative articles are often judged on their authenticity and trustworthiness, rather than validity or reliability (see Figure 8.1, which provides a more detailed explanation).

Appraising the quality of articles is crucial, as it allows for the exploration of how differences in quality might explain differences in the study results. It also guides the interpretation of the findings and their value for practice. Numerous practical issues need to be considered when appraising a study (CRD 2009). These include stating who will be assessing the quality of the studies, how many reviewers will be involved, what checklist or scale will be used for quality assessment and how the reviewers will resolve disagreements. Involvement of a colleague or a supervisor is important (if possible) to ensure that all articles are appropriately critiqued. Table 8.1 shows the common features of research critique frameworks for both quantitative and qualitative studies.

Table 8.1 Common features of research critique frameworks

Quantitative	Qualitative
Research design	Philosophical background
Experimental hypothesis	Research design
Operational definitions	Concepts
Population	Context
Sample	Sample
Sampling	Sampling
Validity/reliability of data collection	Auditability of data collection
Data analysis	Credibility/confirmability of data analysis
Generalizability	Transferability

Source: Reprinted from Caldwell, K., Henshaw, L. and Taylor, G. (2011) Developing a framework for critiquing health research: an early evaluation. *Nurse Education Today* 31 (8): e1–7, with permission from Elsevier.

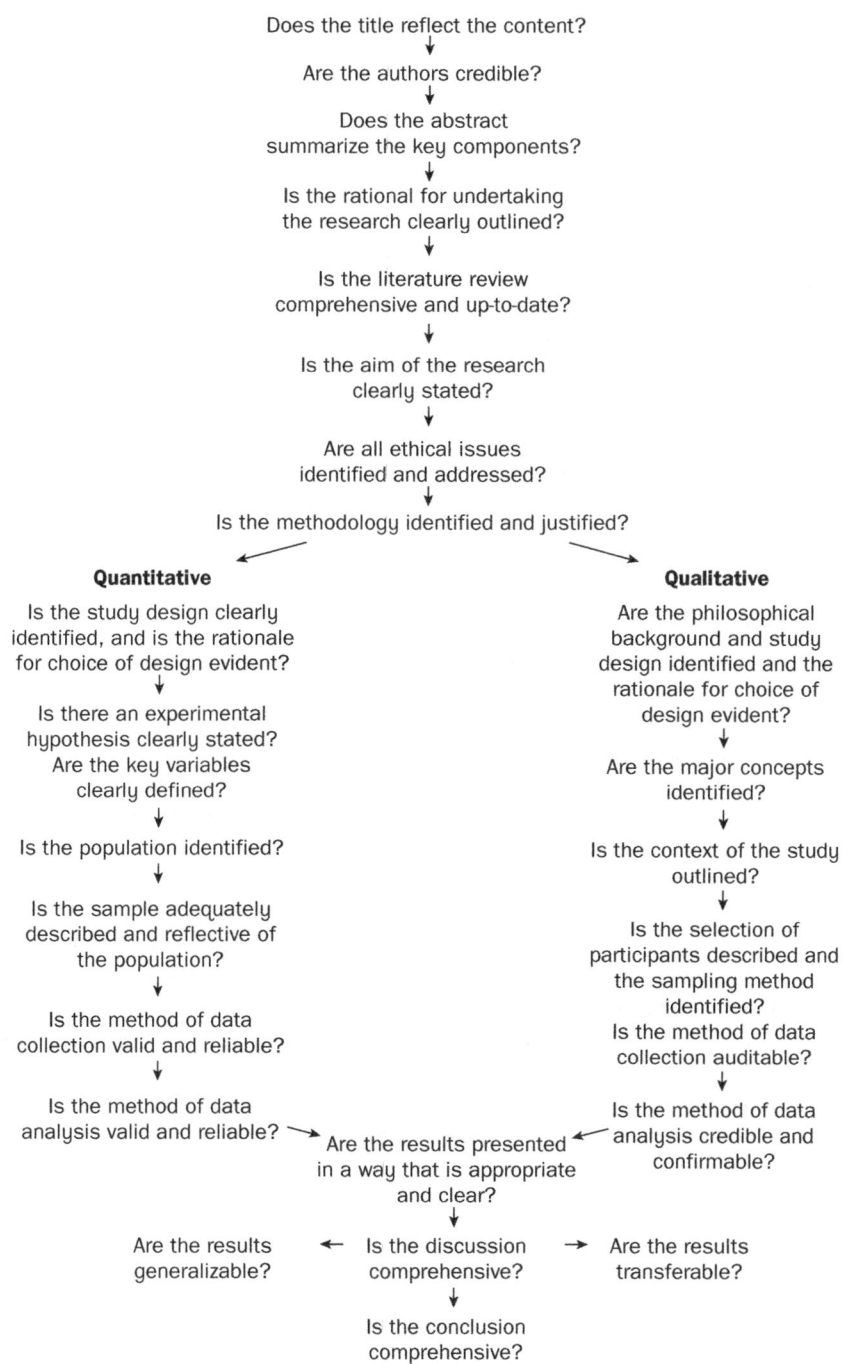

Figure 8.1 Framework by Caldwell et al. (2011).

Source: Reprinted from Caldwell, K., Henshaw, L. and Taylor, G. (2011) Developing a framework for critiquing health research: an early evaluation. *Nurse Education Today* 31 (8): e1–7, with permission from Elsevier.

Another framework, developed by Caldwell et al. (2011) for nursing students, has combined both quantitative and qualitative appraisal questions into one form that can be used for any type of research design. The framework comes with some guidelines that give an explanation of each item. Nursing students have found this framework (Figure 8.1) together with the guidelines (some of which are given here) both easy to use and to follow.

The quality of evidence and conclusions generated by a systematic literature review for nursing practice *depends entirely on the quality of the primary studies that make up the review*. This quality assessment is a key feature that sets apart a systematic review from a narrative review. To assess the quality of primary articles, there are a large selection of assessment or critical appraisal tools that are easily accessible online (see CanChild's critical review forms and guidelines in Box 8.2 later in this chapter). It is important to use appropriate checklists or scales for the type of study design to be evaluated. Box 8.2 lists a number of scales that can be used to evaluate randomized and non-randomized studies, as well as websites where critical appraisal forms for different study designs can be found.

Some useful information on undertaking both quantitative and qualitative critiques can be found in Melnyk and Fineout-Overholt (2018) and Craig and Smyth (2007).

Box 8.2   Websites for some common appraisal frameworks

- The Critical Appraisal Skills Programme, available at http://www.casp-uk.net/ (accessed 12 January 2024)
- CanChild's critical review forms and guidelines, available at https://canchild. ca/en/resources/137-critical-review-forms-and-guidelines (accessed 12 January 2024)
- The Joanna Briggs Institute's critical appraisal tools, available at https://jbi. global/critical-appraisal-tools (accessed 12 January 2024)
- Johns Hopkins University & Medicine. Evidence-based medicine: What is critical appraisal? Available at https://browse.welch.jhmi.edu/EBM/EBM_CriticalAppraisal (accessed 12 January 2024)
- Wells, G.A., Shea, B., O'Connell, D., Peterson, J., Welch, V., Losos, M. and Tugwell, P. (2024) The Newcastle-Ottawa Scale (NOS) for assessing the quality of non-randomized studies in a meta-analysis. Ottawa Hospital. Available at http://www.ohri.ca/programs/clinical_epidemiology/oxford.asp (accessed 12 January 2024)

Practical Tip

Using recognized checklists, scales and/or critical appraisal tools can save you lots of time when undertaking your review. In essence, you do not need to develop these from scratch but can just select the most appropriate tool relevant to your research design. The articles by Buccheri and Sharifi (2017) and Fontaine et al. (2022) detail useful information and resources to support critical appraisal and quality assessment of primary research papers.

One set of critical appraisal forms that we often recommend to students is the McMaster framework for critiquing qualitative or quantitative studies (see Box 8.2). This framework includes excellent guidelines on how to conduct the different kinds of critical appraisals for both quantitative and qualitative research and provides advice for answering each of the questions. Although devised by occupational therapists, the framework is written in basic terms that can be understood by any clinician, researcher or student.

We now return to Caldwell et al.'s (2011) framework, detailed in Figure 8.1. The critical appraisal questions that follow are from Caldwell et al. (2011):

- **Does the title reflect the content?** The title should be informative and indicate the focus of the study. It should allow the reader to easily interpret the content of the study. An inaccurate or misleading title can confuse the reader. Referring back to PICOT (population, intervention, comparative intervention, outcomes and types of studies) and PEOT (population, exposure, outcomes and types of studies), does the title include all these components?

- **Are the authors credible?** Researchers should hold appropriate academic qualifications and be linked to a professional field relevant to the research. Usually at the top of the paper, where the authors names are listed, you will find their qualifications.

- **Does the abstract summarize the key components?** The abstract should provide a short summary of the study. It needs to include the aim of the study, an outline of the methodology and the main findings. The purpose of the abstract is to allow the reader to decide if the study is of interest to them.

- **Is the rationale for undertaking the research clearly outlined?** The author/s need/s to present a clear rationale for the research, placing it in the context of any current issues and knowledge of the topic to date.

- **Is the literature review comprehensive and up to date?** The literature review should reflect the current state of knowledge relevant to the study and identify any gaps or conflicts. It should include key or classic studies on the topic as well as up-to-date literature. There should be a balance of primary and secondary sources.

- **Is the aim of the research clearly stated?** The aim of the study should be clearly stated and should convey what the researcher is setting out to achieve.

- **Are all ethical issues identified and addressed?** Ethical issues pertinent to the study should be discussed. The researcher should identify how the rights of informants have been protected and informed consent obtained. If the research is conducted within the National Health Service (NHS), there should be an indication of approval by a local research ethics committee.

- **Is the methodology identified and justified?** The researcher should make clear which research strategy they are adopting – qualitative or quantitative. A clear rationale for the choice should also be provided, so that the reader can judge whether the chosen strategy is appropriate for the study. At this point the student is asked to look specifically at the questions that apply to the paradigm appropriate to the study they are critiquing.

- **Are the results presented in a way that is appropriate and clear?** Presentation of data should be clear, easily interpretable and consistent.

- **Is the discussion comprehensive?** In quantitative studies the results and discussion are presented separately. In qualitative studies these may be integrated. Whatever the mode of presentation, the researcher should compare and contrast the findings with that of previous research on the topic. The discussion should be balanced and avoid subjectivity.

- **Is the conclusion comprehensive?** Conclusions must be supported by the findings. The researcher should identify any limitations to the study. There may also be recommendations for further research or, if appropriate, implications for practice in the relevant field.

To complete your critique, the final questions that you need to address – applicable to either quantitative or qualitative studies – are outlined in Table 8.2.

The questions posed in Figure 8.1 that are specifically relevant to either quantitative or qualitative research are discussed further below. We have included a worked example using the framework by Caldwell et al. (2011).

Worked example using Caldwell et al.'s (2011) framework to critique a nursing paper

By now you should have familiarized yourself with the questions to ask when critiquing quantitative and/or qualitative papers. Below you will find a worked example of a critique of a research paper taken from the nursing literature. We hope that this will provide a useful illustration of how to critique a paper. We also feel this may help you to think through the issues that need to be considered to comprehensively critique a paper appropriately.

The title of the paper is 'Biofeedback intervention for stress and anxiety among nursing students: A randomized controlled trial' and it is available at https://www.ncbi.nlm.nih.gov/pmc/articles/PMC3395228/ (accessed 12 January 2024). This paper was written by P. Ratanasiripong, N. Ratanasiripong and D. Kathalae and published in *International Scholarly Research Network (ISRN) Nursing*, volume 2012, with article ID 827972, and it is five pages long. See Table 8.3 for a critique of the paper.

Actions during and following the completion of your critique

An important point to remember is that you should score the various questions while you are doing your critique. Once you have completed the critique you need to provide a holistic assessment of whether the quality of this paper was excellent, high, medium, low or very low. The lowest score is 1 and the highest is 3 for each individual question. You then need to total the scores for each question, providing a total score for the paper. For this paper a score of 26/36 was achieved, indicating that the quality of the paper could have been improved – in other words, there were many errors. In research terms this could be stated as a significant amount of bias found within the study. (Please refer to Chapter 10 for further discussion.)

Table 8.2 Questions specifically relevant to either quantitative or qualitative research

Quantitative	Qualitative
Is the design clearly identified and a rationale provided? The design of the study, e.g. a survey experiment, should be identified and justified. As with the choice of strategy, the reader needs to determine whether the design is appropriate for the research undertaken.	*Are the philosophical background and study design identified and the rationale for choice evident?* The design of the study – e.g. phenomenology, ethnography, etc. – should be identified and the philosophical background and rationale discussed. The reader needs to consider if it is appropriate to meet the aims of the study.
Is there an experimental hypothesis clearly stated and are the key variables identified? In experimental research, the researcher should provide a hypothesis. This should clearly identify the independent and dependent variables and state their relationship and the intent of the study. In survey research the researcher may choose to provide a hypothesis, but it is not essential; alternatively, a research question or aim may be provided.	*Are the major concepts identified?* The researchers should make clear what the major concepts are, but they might not define them. The purpose of the study is to explore the concepts from the perspective of the participants.
Is the population identified? The population is the total number of units from which the researcher can gather data. It may be individuals, organizations or documentation. Whatever the unit, it must be clearly identified.	*Is the context of the study outlined?* The researcher should provide a description of the context of the study, how the study sites were determined and how the participants were selected.
Is the sample adequately described and reflective of the population? Both the method of sampling and the size of the sample should be stated so that the reader can judge whether the sample is representative of the population and sufficiently large to eliminate bias.	*Is the selection of the participants described and sampling method identified?* Informants are selected for their relevant knowledge or experience. Representativeness is not a criterion and purposive sampling is often used. Sample size may be determined through saturation.
Is the method of data collection valid and reliable? The process of data collection should be described. The tools or instruments must be appropriate to the aims of the study and the researcher should identify how reliability and validity were assured.	*Is the method of data collection auditable?* Data collection methods should be described and should be appropriate for the aims of the study. The researcher should describe how they assured that the method is auditable.
Is the method of data analysis valid and reliable? The method of data analysis must be described and justified. Any statistical test used should be appropriate for the data involved.	*Is the method of data analysis credible and confirmable?* The data analysis strategy should be identified – what processes were used to identify patterns and themes? The researcher should identify how credibility and confirmability have been addressed.

Source: Reprinted from Caldwell, K., Henshaw, L. and Taylor, G. (2011) Developing a framework for critiquing health research: an early evaluation. *Nurse Education Today* 31 (8): e1–7, with permission from Elsevier.

173

Practice session 8.1

Once you have read through the framework and guidelines (see Figure 8.1), work through the appropriate questions for your type of paper (qualitative or quantitative) and try to critique them. Alternatively, you can select either the quantitative or the qualitative critical appraisal forms available on any of the various websites provided in Box 8.2.

🔑 Key points

- A quality assessment of your primary research papers is one of the key features that sets apart a systematic review from a narrative review.
- To assess the quality of your primary research papers, there are a number of assessment or critical appraisal tools that are easily accessible online, or you can use the framework by Caldwell et al. (2011), included in this chapter.
- It is important to use an appropriate checklist or scales that are designed specifically for the type of study design that you are evaluating. You may have to use more than one type of critical appraisal tool, depending on the type of research design you are reviewing.

Summary

This chapter discussed the second main stage involved in working with your primary research papers. It has detailed the importance of appraising the methodological quality of your articles and included useful tools and frameworks to aid you in the process. The importance of using a form or framework to standardize and increase the reliability and validity for all stages of the process was clarified by using relevant examples from nursing practice.

Question and Answer (Q&A)

(Q) Is there any one critical appraisal framework available that I should use to review the primary research papers that have been found during the literature search, the initial screening of title and abstracts, and the full-paper screening?

(A) There are numerous critical appraisal frameworks available to aid you with your quality assessment. Prior to undertaking the quality assessment we would suggest that you follow some of links provided in this chapter to read up on the various frameworks. In our experience, a good way to establish which one is best for you is to review and complete these before you commence your systematic review. In this chapter we have highlighted and discussed Caldwell et al.'s (2011) framework. This can be used to appraise both quantitative and qualitative methods.

Table 8.3 Worked example of a critique using Caldwell et al.'s (2011) framework questions for the paper 'Biofeedback intervention for stress and anxiety among nursing students: A randomized controlled trial'

	Framework questions (Caldwell et al. 2011)	Evaluation	Score
1	Does the title reflect the content?	Yes, the title of this paper is reflective of the content of the paper. The PICO components are clearly stated as well as the research design of the study (RCT). Although the comparative intervention is not included in the title it is clear that there must be a comparative intervention, as the research design is an RCT. However, it is unclear from the title what the comparative intervention is. It is also unclear from the title what specific biofeedback machine was used.	1
2	Are the authors credible?	Although the professional titles and the qualifications of the authors cannot be found in the paper, the fact that all three authors' addresses are university addresses suggests that they are lecturers or assistant professors with appropriate qualifications. It would have been helpful, however, for the editor/s of the journal to have included the qualifications of the authors to enable readers to better appraise the authors' credibility.	1,
3	Does the abstract summarize the key components?	Yes, the abstract provided for this paper includes a structured abstract with subheadings, so the purpose, methods, results and conclusions are very clear. It is unclear from the abstract, however, what the specific biofeedback device is.	1
4	Is the rationale for undertaking the research clearly outlined?	Yes, this was clearly explained by describing what previous studies had and had not investigated (i.e. the gap in the literature was clearly highlighted). The authors stated that no recent studies had been conducted with the new generation of portable biofeedback equipment that addressed nursing students' stress and anxiety; however, the reader is left to take this statement at face value without being clear as to how comprehensive and how in-depth the search for papers was.	2
5	Is the literature review comprehensive and up to date?	The authors have thoroughly described previous studies in the area and the papers appear to be up to date.	2

(continued)

175

Table 8.3 Continued

	Framework questions (Caldwell et al. 2011)	Evaluation	Score
6	Is the aim of the study clearly stated?	The purpose is clearly described in the abstract; however, it does not seem to be restated within the main paper after the background section.	2
7	Are all ethical issues identified and addressed?	Yes, all ethical issues appear to have been identified and addressed. The study was approved by the nursing college's institutional review board for ethical approval and all participants in the study volunteered to take part and signed the informed consent forms.	2
8	Is the methodology identified and addressed?	Yes, the methodology was very clearly identified and addressed.	1
9	Is the design clearly identified and a rationale provided?	Yes, the research design was appropriately identified as an RCT but a rationale was not provided.	1
10	Is an experimental hypothesis clearly stated and are the key variables identified?	No, the experimental hypothesis was not specifically stated, but the purpose of the study was very clearly stated. However, as stated in Table 8.2, it is not essential to do this for surveys. The key variables were not explicitly stated; however, both the independent variable (the biofeedback intervention) and the dependent variables (stress and anxiety) were described in depth.	1
11	Is the population identified?	Yes, the population was clearly identified. It consisted of 60 second-year baccalaureate nursing students aged between 18 and 21 years.	2
12	Is the sample adequately described and reflective of the population?	Yes, both the method of sampling and the size of the sample were clearly described so the reader could judge that the sample was representative of the population and sufficiently large to eliminate bias. In fact, the authors also calculated an a priori power analysis that identified that at least 60 participants were needed.	2

(continued)

Table 8.3 Continued

	Framework questions (Caldwell et al. 2011)	Evaluation	Score
13	Is the method of data collection valid and reliable?	Yes, the method of data collection appeared to be valid and reliable with some exceptions; it was unclear precisely how the participants were randomly allocated to the biofeedback or the comparison intervention (i.e. nothing). This could have led to allocation bias. Additionally the instrument should have been clearly described in a separate instrumentation section that needed to be located before the procedure section. The internal consistency of both the anxiety and stress scales were discussed. It is unclear, however, whether the reliability of the biofeedback device was assessed.	1
14	Is the method of data analysis valid and reliable? The method of data analysis must be described and justified. Any statistical test used should be appropriate for the data involved.	The method of data analysis was described and justified. However, more appropriate tests could have been selected to enhance the validity of the study. The statistical tests used were adequate for the data involved but involved conducting more tests than necessary, which could have led to a type 1 error (this is where the results indicate that the intervention is effective when in reality it is not). For example, a more appropriate test that would have assessed all the differences between the four areas below could have been applied:

1. Pre-intervention biofeedback and comparative group
2. Post-intervention biofeedback and comparison group
3. Differences between the pre- and post-biofeedback data
4. Differences between the pre- and post-comparative intervention data.

In this instance the most appropriate statistical test (assuming the data were normally distributed) would have been a two-way ANOVA with repeated measures and a post hoc test. A statistically significant ANOVA test lets you know that there are significant differences between different groups, but it does not let you know specifically which groups are significantly different, so that is why you need a post hoc test. Usually this is either the Bonferroni test or the Tukey post hoc test. | 1 |

(continued)

Table 8.3 Continued

Framework questions (Caldwell et al. 2011)	Evaluation	Score
15 Are the results presented in a way that is appropriate and clear?	Yes, the results were presented very clearly through the use of graphs and tables that were clearly labelled and explained within the text. Good use was made of colour to differentiate between the biofeedback and the comparison groups.	2
16 Is the discussion comprehensive?	Partly.	1
17 Is the conclusion comprehensive?	Yes, the conclusions were comprehensive. The limitations of the study were clearly discussed, as were the implications for nursing practice. Recommendations were appropriately made for further research in this field.	2
18 Are the results generalizable?	Yes and no. The results are definitely generalizable to other nursing schools within Thailand, but we do not know if they are generalizable to nursing schools in different countries, as these were not included within the study. However, the assumption is that the results would be generalizable to nursing schools in other countries.	1
		26/36

References

Buccheri, R.K. and Sharifi, C. (2017) Critical appraisal tools and reporting guidelines for evidence-based practice. *Worldviews on Evidence-Based Nursing* 14 (6): 463–472.

Caldwell, K., Henshaw, L. and Taylor, G. (2011) Developing a framework for critiquing health research: An early evaluation. *Nurse Education Today* 31 (8): e1–7.

Craig, J.V. and Smyth, R.L. (2007) *The Evidence-Based Practice Manual for Nurses*, 2nd edn. London: Churchill Livingstone.

CRD (Centre for Reviews and Dissemination) (2009) *Systematic Reviews: CRD's Guidance for Undertaking Reviews in Health Care*. Available at http://www.york.ac.uk/crd/guidance/ (accessed 12 January 2024).

Fontaine, G., Maheu-Cadotte, M.A., Lavallée, A. et al. (2022) Designing, planning, and conducting systematic reviews and other knowledge syntheses: Six key practical recommendations to improve feasibility and efficiency. *Worldviews on Evidence-Based Nursing* 19 (6): 434–441.

Higgins, J.P.T., Thomas, J., Chandler, J. et al. (eds) (2023) *Cochrane Handbook for Systematic Reviews of Interventions*, version 6.4 (updated August 2023). Available at www.training. cochrane.org/handbook (accessed 24 November 2023).

Jadad, A. (1998) *Randomized Controlled Trials: A User's Guide*. London: BMJ Books.

Melnyk, B.M. and Fineout-Overholt, E. (2018) *Evidence-Based Practice in Nursing and Healthcare: A Guide to Best Practice*, 4th edn. Philadelphia, PA: Wolters Kluwer.

Texas A&M University (2024) Nursing research guide: Experimental design and RCTs: A research guide for students in the College of Nursing and Health Sciences. Available at https://guides. library.tamucc.edu/c.php?g=895836&p=6497167 (accessed 10 January 2024).

9

Working with your primary papers: Stage 3 – Extracting the data from your included papers

Overview

- Extracting the appropriate data from the chosen research papers
- The process of data extraction as applied to Mary's quantitative systematic review on domestic violence
- The process of data extraction as applied to Sue's qualitative systematic review on witnessed resuscitation
- The process of data extraction as applied to Fay's quantitative systematic review on sterile versus non-sterile catheter insertion

Extracting the appropriate data from your research papers

The methods section of your review needs to cover the three stages detailed in Box 9.1. This chapter details Stage 3, focusing on how to extract the right data from the primary research papers you have selected. This will enable you to answer your systematic review question.

Box 9.1   Methods of the review

In this section you need to give details of the following three separate stages:

Stage 1: The process of selecting the papers for inclusion in the systematic review. This stage has two steps (see Chapter 7).

Stage 2: The process for the assessment of methodological quality (see Chapter 8).

Stage 3: The process for the proposed data extraction strategy.

The data extraction phase is perhaps the most challenging aspect of the systematic review process. Data extraction involves going back to the primary research articles and highlighting the relevant information that will answer your systematic review question. Normally, this involves extracting data related to the population included, the intervention, comparative intervention, outcomes and research design (the PICOT components). To standardize this process and improve the validity of the results, it is crucial for you to compile a data extraction form. As with the selection form previously described, it is important to pilot the form on one or two of the selected primary research articles to ensure it is useful and appropriate (Büchter et al. 2020; Büchter et al. 2023; Higgins et al. 2023). Examples of the forms and how these can be applied in practice are provided in Mary's, Sue's and Fay's case studies detailed below.

The process of data extraction as applied to Mary's quantitative systematic review on domestic violence

Ⓜ Let us first consider the example of Mary's quantitative study on domestic violence. Mary needs to look back at the PICOT form she made when selecting her articles, presented in Chapter 7 (see Tables 7.1 and 7.2). She knows that all the articles included in the final selection are relevant to the research question and have met the inclusion criteria. In the data extraction form, it is important that she extracts all the relevant information to enable her to answer her review question related to women who have suffered from domestic violence. As well as collecting information on the study design, population, intervention and control group, Mary will need to collect information on the outcomes. Table 9.1 provides an example of what one of Mary's data extraction forms might look like, together with our comments on what Mary needs to do in each section.

Ⓜ **Table 9.1** An example of what Mary's data extraction form could look like

Date of data extraction: 23/4/11 *(here Mary writes down the date when she fills in the form)*

Reviewer: Mary Smith *(here she writes her name as the reviewer of the paper)*

Bibliographic details of study: *(here she writes the reference for the paper)*

Jones, J. (2008) The effect of advocacy interventions compared to usual care on abused women's quality of life. *Journal of Clinical Nursing* 10 (5): 345–352.

Purpose of study: *(here she writes down the purpose of the paper from which she is extracting the data)*

The purpose of the study is to evaluate the effectiveness of a community advocacy programme, as compared with usual care, in terms of abused women's quality of life (QOL).

Study design: *(here she writes down the study design – usually this can be found in the abstract)*

Randomized controlled trial (RCT)

Population (sample): *(here she summarizes the information about the sample used in the paper)*

Sixty women who were experiencing or had previously experienced domestic violence were included in the study. The women were randomly allocated to either the intervention group (*n*=30) or the control group, who received usual care (*n*=30).

Intervention: *(Mary summarizes what the intervention was)*

Women attended an advocacy group once a week over 12 weeks. Group meetings provided support and help for women on all aspects relevant to domestic violence.

Comparative intervention: *(the same for the comparative intervention)*

The women in this group received usual care.

(continued)

Table 9.1 (continued)

Outcomes: *(This part is very important. Mary needs to search for the results of each primary research study in the results section of each primary research article. As her outcomes relate to QOL scales she needs to copy the pre- and post-intervention values for both the advocacy group and the usual care group, as seen below. In this case the results of this paper have been extracted)*

SF-36 QOL scales

Pre-intervention advocacy group 30/50 (50 is the average rate for healthy individuals)

Post-intervention advocacy group 40/50

Pre-intervention usual care group 29/50

Post-intervention usual care group 30/50

The process of data extraction as applied to Sue's qualitative systematic review on witnessed resuscitation

Ⓢ Turning to Sue's qualitative systematic literature review, Sue first needs to make a data extraction form to extract relevant data for the data extraction process. This part of the process is identical whether you are planning to extract qualitative or quantitative data. The key difference between the two types of data extraction forms (qualitative or quantitative) is that the outcomes section in a qualitative data extraction form will be inserted under the main themes that were decided upon for your systematic review question when you were planning your protocol or plan; the data extracted will be in the form of 'words or perceptions' of the population group(s) you have decided to include. For quantitative data extraction forms, it is mostly numbers that are extracted.

Sue has decided to include three different population groups, as listed in Box 9.2. When constructing the outcomes section of her data extraction form, she also needs to include a section where she will write down the page number, column number and line numbers of the words extracted (sentences and paragraphs that she will extract from her included primary research papers). This will let her know what part of the paper the excerpt came from and improve the audit trail of her systematic review. Table 9.2 provides an example of what Sue's data extraction form looked like before she filled it in.

Ⓢ Box 9.2   Sue's proposed outcomes

- Outcome 1: Patients' experiences of resuscitation and/or invasive procedures (Table 9.3)
- Outcome 2: Family members' experiences of resuscitation and/or invasive procedures (Table 9.4)
- Outcome 3: Healthcare professionals' (HCPs') experiences of resuscitation and/or invasive procedures (Table 9.5)

§ **Table 9.2** Sample of Sue's data extraction form

Date of data extraction:	*(Today's date)*
Reviewer:	*(Your name)*
Bibliographical details of study:	*(Full reference of article including author, year and source)*
Purpose of study:	*(This is outlined by the author of the article)*
Study design:	*(Type of qualitative study utilized for purpose of the article)*
Population (sample):	*(This section outlines the description of the study sample characteristics as identified)*
Number: **Age:** **Ethnicity:** **Exposure:**	*(Witnessed resuscitation and/or invasive procedures)*

Having completed the data extraction, it is important to highlight and summarize the outcomes. Examples of how to capture and present the outcomes of Sue's case study are provided in Tables 9.3 to 9.5.

§ **Table 9.3** Outcome 1: Patients' experiences of resuscitation and/or invasive procedures

Page	Col.	Line	Data extracted	Sub-themes

§ **Table 9.4** Outcome 2: Family members' experiences of resuscitation and/or invasive procedures

Page of paper	Col.	Line	Data extracted	Sub-themes

§ **Table 9.5** Outcome 3: HCPs' experiences of resuscitation and/or invasive procedures

Page	Col.	Line	Data extracted	Sub-themes

Once the data extraction form is ready, Sue can proceed with the data extraction process. There are several approaches to extracting data from qualitative papers, with no one way being more popular than others. There is an emerging evidence base within the literature providing examples of data extraction and coding information templates along with the various analysis tools and frameworks. Figure 9.1 provides more information.

Practical Tip

Before starting your review it is important to look at examples of how other researchers have developed their own qualitative data extraction forms. You may find the article by Davies (2019) useful in guiding you through this aspect of your systematic review.

Below we have outlined three ways of extracting data from your primary research studies but there are many different ways this can be done. Some other examples are presented in Figure 9.1, and further qualitative data analysis approaches are available in Busetto et al. (2020).

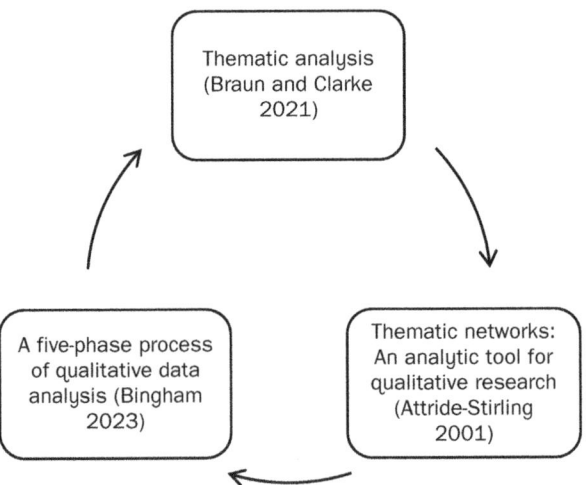

Figure 9.1 Qualitative data analysis approaches.

The method described below has been adapted from Burnard's (1991) method of thematic analysis and follows the same methodology that you would use to review any qualitative data, for example interviews. Burnard (1991) has published an excellent detailed description of the steps involved in his article entitled 'A method of analysing interview transcripts in qualitative research'. In the next part of this chapter, you will find a description for one process for extracting data from a research paper. Below we take you through each step of the processes.

Step 1

Before Sue starts extracting qualitative data (i.e. words and sentences) it is important that she reads the *results section* of her primary papers a number of times in order to become fully immersed in the data. The purpose of immersion is to become more fully aware of the 'lived world' of the participants and to try to see the world from the other person's perspective.

 ### Step 2

As part of her review question Sue has decided which specific themes she intends to look at as part of developing her review question. Sue is looking at the perspectives of three different population groups – the patients, the families and the HCPs – and has colour-coded them in three different colours. Sue's colour-coding scheme involves highlighting any perceptions in the primary research papers to do with patients in green, any families' perceptions in yellow and any HCPs' perspectives in blue. This can be done either manually by using highlighter pens or electronically on a computer.

 ### Step 3

The next step is to cut out (either manually or electronically) all the text highlighted in different colours and paste it in the 'Data extracted' section of the form. In Sue's scenario, all green highlighted text related to patients will be inserted under Outcome 1 of the form, all yellow highlighted text related to family members will be inserted under Outcome 2 of the form and all blue highlighted text under Outcome 3. Eventually Sue will end up with all the data or text in the primary paper related to patients, family members and HCPs under the appropriate headings and sections in the data extraction form (see Table 9.2). She also needs to make sure that she notes down the page number, column number and line number from the primary paper, as she will need this information when she refers to the data in the results or discussion sections of her review. It is important to clarify your audit trail.

 ### Step 4

In the data extraction form, Sue writes down as many headings as necessary to describe all aspects of the content excluding 'dross'. Field and Morse (1985) state that the term 'dross' is used to denote any unusable fillers in an interview or paper, such as issues that are unrelated to the topic at hand. The headings or category system should account for almost all the category data. This phase is known as *open coding*, meaning that categories are generated freely (Burnard 1991: 462).

 ### Step 5

When Sue has written down all the categories for the results section, the next step is for her to look through the headings and to try to group them together under higher-order headings. Burnard (1991) explains that the aim here is to reduce the number of categories by collapsing some of the ones that are similar into broader categories. For example, it could be decided that all the headings in the 'categories' column could be collapsed into one higher-order heading as shown in Table 9.6.

Table 9.6 HCPs' experiences of resuscitation and/or invasive procedures

Outcome/theme 3

HCPs' experiences of resuscitation and/or invasive procedures					Higher-order headings
Page	Col.	Line	Data extracted	Open coding	Categories	

(table content)

Page	Col.	Line	Data extracted	Open coding	Categories	Higher-order headings
90	1	35–39	Other concerns stemmed from the insertion of chest drains, defibrillating, putting in tubes, inserting needles and intubation	Concerns arising from insertion of diverse medical devices	HCPs' concerns relating to family's needs	HCPs' concerns for family needs and feelings during the procedure
91	1	1–3	All of these are invasive procedures that are 'abnormal in their (the relatives') eyes, and therefore difficult for the relatives to witness'	Invasive procedures / Abnormal procedures for relatives / Difficult for families to witness	Invasive and abnormal procedures / HCPs' concern for families' feelings	

Step 6

The new list of categories are worked through and very similar headings are removed.

Step 7

This step is used to 'increase the validity of the categorizing method and to guard against researcher bias' (Burnard 1991: 463). It is important to ask one or two colleagues to independently generate the categories from the same research paper without looking at your own list. Once this has been done the categories are discussed and any changes made as necessary.

Step 8

When you have obtained a revised list, you will need to reread the results section of the research paper and make sure that the final categories and subheadings still cover *all the relevant parts* of the results section. Then make any changes you think necessary.

Step 9

Once this has been done for one primary research paper, the same process is carried out for all the included papers. One of Sue's completed data extraction forms is shown in Table 9.7. The process of synthesizing the data extraction forms will be discussed in Chapter 10.

---

§ **Table 9.7** One of Sue's completed data extraction forms

Date of data extraction: 19 March 2011
Reviewer: SH
Bibliographical details of study: Goodenough, T. J. and Brysiewicz, P. (2003) Witnessed resuscitation: Exploring the attitudes and practices of the emergency staff working in Level I emergency departments in the province of KwaZulu-Natal. *Curationis* 29 (2): 59–93 (supplied by the British Library).
Area: KwaZulu-Natal
Purpose of study: To explore the attitudes and practices of witnessed resuscitation by the staff working in Level I emergency departments in the province of KwaZulu-Natal
Study design: Qualitative survey
Setting: Emergency departments
Population:
Sample selection: Purposeful sample of six staff members from two different Level I emergency departments. From each of these hospitals the sample consisted of one medical officer, one registered nurse and one registered nurse in charge of the unit. All participants had to have been employed in the department for more than six months in order to ensure they had experienced resuscitation procedures. This purposeful selection method was appropriate to the purpose and question as it identified a combination of attitudes from both clinical and managerial staff.
Number: Six
Length of experience: Minimum 9 months to 8 years
Exposure: Resuscitation/invasive procedures
Outcome/theme 1: Patients' experiences of resuscitation and/or invasive procedures

92	1	1–10	When family members were present the patients felt loved, supported and less alone. One said, 'It would have been awful to be there alone and have no family there by your side. It would be even worse.' Patients recounted that family members hugged and kissed them, held their hands, and listened to their fears. One patient undergoing a lumbar puncture said: 'I was scared that it was going to hurt. I didn't want people going in my back. I was afraid. Having him [a relative] there was so comforting.'	Family presence Comfort measures Reassurance from family members

(Continued overleaf)

§ **Table 9.7** Continued

| 91 | 1 | 22–28 | Patients described themselves as being 'afraid, hurt, and in pain' during the emergency event. They related feeling safer and less scared when family members were there.
'The injuries were so severe ... you can deal with a situation like that a lot better if you have the reinforcement of a loved one.'
'I was very scared. I thought I would never have a leg again. It was broken really badly. I thought I might die. I remember waking up and seeing all those doctors. I was like, Where am I? Something is wrong! I looked over and saw my dad and my mother. They were there to help me, to hold my hand, to give me a hug.' | Family presence Comfort measures Reassurance from parents' presence |

Outcome/theme 2: Family members' experiences of resuscitation and/or invasive procedures

Page	Col.	Line	Data extracted	Subthemes
59	2	20–21	'I couldn't not have been there, I needed to be with him and I was.' (Fran)	Family needs
59	2	23–28	'I felt useful during the event, I genuinely felt that I was contributing positively and that helps me a lot [pauses]. I can also recall that his eyes were looking at me, as though he knew it was me next to him . . . I was able to keep speaking to him – comforting him – I think!' (Jane)	Feeling conscious of presence Feeling useful during event
59	2	35–39	'John didn't know I was there, of course, he can't remember anything of the event for a good two weeks after ... And, I didn't think at the time he would know that I was there. I just stood at the foot of his bed ...' (Ann)	Family needs Familiarity and support for patient

Outcome/theme 3: HCPs' experiences of resuscitation and or invasive procedures

Page	Col.	Line	Data extracted	Sub-themes
90 91	1 1	35–39 1–3	Other concerns stemmed from the insertion of chest drains, defibrillating, putting in tubes, inserting needles and intubation. All of these are invasive procedures that are 'abnormal in their (the relatives') eyes, and therefore difficult for the relatives to witness.'	Family needs Concern for families' feelings

(Continued overleaf)

§ **Table 9.7** Continued

Page	Col.	Line	Data extracted	Sub-themes
90	2	29–31	The staff didn't think that the relatives should be present at the resuscitation of their loved one, and they said they would prefer not to be present at the resuscitation of their own family members. 'I totally disagree with allowing family members into the resuscitation room ...' 'I don't think it's very nice.'	Family needs Concern for families' feelings

When Sue has extracted her data from one paper, she needs to repeat the process for all her included studies. Sue's data should now be synthesized, which means putting it all together or combining it. This is usually carried out by using tables or graphics for quantitative data or presenting them under themes for qualitative data. The ways of doing this will be discussed in Chapter 10.

F One of Fay's completed data extraction forms can be seen below in Figure 9.2.

CAUTI: Sterile Versus Non-sterile Catheter Insertion

DATA Extraction Form

Details of Study 8:

TITLE: Comparison of a Microbicidal Povidone-iodine gel and a placebo gel as catheter lubricants. (Author: Harrison, L H. (1980))
SOURCE: *The Journal of Urology,* 124 (3):pq 347–349.

Reviewer's Name: Fiona Bezzina   Date: 6th Sept 2008

Purpose of the study: to evaluate the Microbicidal effect and lubricating action of Povidone-iodine lubricating gel when used clinically as a catheter lubricant. Patient acceptance and tolerance, burning or stinging sensation, were also recorded.

Study Design: Cohort study

POPULATION:

Sample size: 50 (intervention group n=26; control group n=24)

Criteria of diagnosis (CAUTI or Bacteriuria): Urethral bacterial colony counts

Any Secondary diagnosis: Urinary Tract and/or Prostatic disorders

Inclusion/Exclusion Criteria: No information given on the inclusion criteria.
Exclusion criteria: Patients who were known to be sensitive to the ingredients of the test or the control gels; subjects who were on antibiotics and patients suffering from urethral burning, stinging or irritation or any medical problem requiring treatment that might have interfered with the results.

CAUTI: Sterile Versus Non-sterile Catheter Insertion

Study 8: Harrison (1980)   Data Extraction Form (Continued)

Type of Catheterisation: urethral, Intermittent and indwelling
Reason for catheterisation: Urinary tract or prostatic disorders
Setting: Nor clearly stated; probably in hospital.

INTERVENTION:

Experimental Intervention/s: Penis was held by an attendant and the glans was rinsed with sterile distilled water. Distal urethral swab was taken. Using sterile technique, povidone iodine gel was applied along the length of the catheter which was then inserted. Patient was asked about subjective sensation (burning or stinging sensation). 3 minutes post-insertion the catheter was withdrawn and another swab was taken from the portion of the catheter that previously was in contact with the urethra. All specimens were sent to the microbiology laboratory.
Duration of Intervention/s: 3 Minutes
Adverse Effects: None reported
Control Treatment/s: same protocol as experimental but K-Y jelly was used as lubricant.

Drop-outs: None reported

OUTCOMES:

CAUTI:

    Number of UTI's (in Experimental and Control groups):

        Bacteriuria (Urine sample):
        Symptomatic UTI:
        Combined Results:

> The pre-catheterisation geometric mean (the average of the logarithim counts) was 9549.9 for the Povidone-iodine gel group and 7244.4 for controls. Post-catheterisation values were 44.7 and 658.2, respectively.

    Types of Infecting Organisms:
        Staphylococcus, Streptococcus, Enterococcus,

    Time of Urine Sample/UTI (from Catheter insertion):
        Bacterial count at 3 minutes post-catheterisation

CAUTI Incidence Rate (as percentage) in:

    Intervention Group:

    Control Group:

    Statistical significance:

> Bacterial count reduction achieved with Povidone-iodine lubricating gel was significantly greater than achieved with the control lubricating gel.
> Statistical analysis, using the Mann-Whitney U-test, giving the value of $p<0.02$

UTI Rate according to Gender: All male subjects

Figure 9.2 Fay's completed data extraction form.

Practice session 9.1

Below we have included a number of templates that you might want to use for your own data extraction (Boxes 9.3 to 9.7).

Box 9.3   Template to use for quantitative generic data extraction

Details of study 1 (bibliographical reference):

Title:

Source:

Purpose of the study:

Reviewer's name: Date:

Study design:

Population:

Sample size:

Criteria of diagnosis:

Any secondary diagnosis:

Exclusion criteria:

Setting:

Intervention:

Comparative intervention:

Outcomes:

Adverse effects:

Box 9.4   Template to use for qualitative generic data extraction

Date of data extraction:

Reviewer:

Bibliographical details of study:

Purpose of study:

Study design:

Setting:

Population:

Sample selection:

Number:

Age:

Education, years:

Ethnicity/race:

Religion:

Relationship of family member:

Primary diagnosis at time of event:

Exposure:

Box 9.5   Outcomes: theme 1

Population experiences 1

Page	Col.	Line	Data extracted	Subthemes

Box 9.6   Outcomes: theme 2

Population experiences 2

Page	Col.	Line	Data extracted	Subthemes

Box 9.7   Outcomes: theme 3

Population experiences 3

Page	Col.	Line	Data extracted	Subthemes

Key points

- Data extraction involves going back to the primary research articles (mostly the results section) and highlighting the relevant information that will serve to answer the research question.
- This involves extracting data related to the population included, the intervention, the comparative group, the outcomes and the research design (the PICOT components).
- To standardize this process and improve the validity of the results, it is crucial to compile a data extraction form specific to your systematic review question.

Summary

This chapter discussed the third stage of the methods of the systematic review, associated with how to extract the appropriate qualitative and quantitative data from your primary research papers. The importance of using a form or framework to standardize and increase the reliability and validity for all stages of the process was clarified by using relevant examples from nursing practice.

Question and Answer (Q&A)

(Q) Are there any standardized data extraction forms or frameworks available to aid with data extraction for both quantitative and qualitative reviews?

(A) There are several data extraction framework examples available on the internet (such as on systematic review websites) as well as in numerous research methods books. However, a data extraction form is generally designed according to a very specific systematic review question. Looking at other data extraction forms, both in your specific area and in other areas (for example on the internet or in other students' dissertations), may help you with the general design of your own data extraction form. We would also recommend that prior to commencing your own systematic review, you explore what is available in the literature (and elsewhere) and then select the most appropriate ways that data extraction tools could help you to complete your own data extraction for your systematic review.

References

Attride-Stirling, J. (2001) Thematic networks: An analytic tool for qualitative research. *Qualitative Research* 1 (3): 385–405.

Bingham, A. J. (2023) From data management to actionable findings: A five-phase process of qualitative data analysis. *International Journal of Qualitative Methods* 22. https://doi.org/10.1177/16094069231183620

Braun, V. and Clarke, V. (2021) *Thematic Analysis: A Practical Guide*. London: Sage.

Büchter, R.B., Weise, A. and Pieper, D. (2020) Development, testing and use of data extraction forms in systematic reviews: A review of methodological guidance. *BMC Medical Research Methodology* 20: 259.

Büchter, B.R., Rombey, T., Mathes, T. et al. (2023) Systematic reviewers used various approaches to data extraction and expressed several research needs: A survey. *Journal of Clinical Epidemiology* 159: 214–224.

Burnard, P. (1991) A method of analysing interview transcripts in qualitative research. *Nurse Education Today* 11 (6): 461–466.

Busetto, L., Wick, W. and Gumbinger, C. (2020) How to use and assess qualitative research methods. *Neurological Research and Practice* 2: Art. 14.

Davies, A. (2019) Carrying out systematic literature reviews: An introduction. *British Journal of Nursing* 8:28 (15): 1008–1014.

Field, P. and Morse, J. (1985) *Nursing Research: The Application of Qualitative Practices*, 2nd edn. London: Croom Helm.

Higgins, J.P.T., Thomas, J., Chandler, J. et al. (eds) (2023) *Cochrane Handbook for Systematic Reviews of Interventions*, version 6.4 (updated August 2023). Available at www.training.cochrane.org/handbook (accessed 24 November 2023).

10

Synthesizing, summarizing and presenting your findings

Overview

- Issues to consider when synthesizing and summarizing your results
- Tools to use when synthesizing and summarizing your results
- How and where to get started on presenting your results
- Presenting the results of your search
- Presenting the results of the studies selected based on the title and abstract
- Presenting the results of the studies selected based on reading the full paper
- Presenting a summary of all your included studies
- Presenting a summary of all the critiques of your included papers using the appropriate frameworks
- Presenting a summary of the data extracted (including a synthesis of the overall results)
- Summarizing, synthesizing and presenting your interventions and comparative interventions
- Summarizing, synthesizing and presenting your outcomes
- Summarizing, synthesizing and presenting quantitative outcome measures
- Summarizing, synthesizing and presenting qualitative outcome measures

Issues to consider when synthesizing and summarizing your results

When synthesizing and summarizing your data, there are several issues that you need to consider. Popay et al. (2006: 6; emphasis in original) state that 'the synthesis, *at a minimum*, is a summary of the current state of knowledge in relation to a particular review question'. This is the section where you will attempt to find the answer to your systematic review question. In a quantitative review, if the results are similar enough – for example if the interventions, designs and outcomes are all alike – it may be possible to conduct a statistical procedure, such as a meta-analysis, to combine the results.

In a qualitative review the combined results of all the included studies can be synthesized under major themes or subthemes. This is sometimes called a meta-synthesis or meta-ethnography. It involves a similar approach to the methods of the qualitative data analysis used in the primary qualitative studies being synthesized (Kim and Chang 2022). The Centre for Reviews and Dissemination (CRD 2009) suggests that irrespective of what type of data you have extracted, it is important to first undertake a narrative synthesis of the results of your findings to help you decide what other methods are appropriate.

Practical Tip

In our opinion this is one of the most exciting parts of the review, as it is where you start finding out the answer to your review question.

Popay et al. (2006: 5) state:

> Narrative synthesis is a form of storytelling ... bringing together evidence in a way that tells a convincing story of why something needs to be done, or needs to be stopped, or why we have no idea whether a long established policy or practice makes a positive difference is one of the ways in which the gap between research, policy and practice can start to be bridged. Telling a trustworthy story is at the heart of narrative synthesis.

Popay et al. (2006) and Tranvåg et al. (2016) provide excellent guidance on synthesizing data and narratives. They also present some specific tools and techniques that can be used when synthesizing your results. Narrative synthesis may be used in several different ways (Popay et al. 2006: 7):

- Before undertaking a specialist approach, such as statistical meta-analysis or meta-ethnography
- Instead of a specialist synthesis approach, because the studies included are insufficiently similar to allow for this
- When the systematic review question dictates the inclusion of a wide range of research designs, including qualitative and quantitative designs.

Recapping briefly what was covered in Chapters 7 to 9, once you have selected your primary research papers, appraised the quality of the papers and extracted the appropriate data, how do you go about synthesizing (or combining) the results? Some of the key points associated with data extraction can be summarized as follows:

- Are the data sufficiently similar?
- Are there caveats (explanations to prevent misinterpretation) that need to be acknowledged?
- Are there any particular trends or themes to inform policy and nursing practice?
- Does the data seem to point in one direction or several?

In many disciplines, such as nursing and the social sciences, the quantitative studies involved are either significantly different or in many cases involve qualitative studies that require different methods of synthesis. Some systematic reviews may also include studies of different designs (mixed methods). Irrespective of the type of systematic review, you will need to undertake some form of summary or synthesis.

We would suggest that the primary aim of the majority of systematic reviews in nursing is to answer questions around some of the following:

- addressing a clinical question or problem
- improving policy and guidance
- changing clinical and/or professional practice
- improving safety for patients and staff
- enhancing quality and outcomes.

From our experiences (as is highlighted in Chapter 12) we have found that many students who have completed a systematic review fail to progress their work by presenting and publishing the findings. We recommend that having undertaken and completed your systematic review, it is important to write up and publish your work. This is so that other nurses can benefit from the findings and recommendations. Depending on whether the systematic review is being conducted for a dissertation or is being written up for journal publication, different results may be presented depending on the submission requirements. Journal articles, Cochrane and the Campbell Collaboration have their own recommendations or criteria for presenting the results.

Tools to use when synthesizing and summarizing your results

There are numerous tools that you can use to summarize, synthesize and present your data. A few of the most common ones are (Popay et al. 2006; University of Toledo 2024):

- textual descriptions, which means written words that everyone is familiar with
- grouping of similar data, for example tabulation (presenting the results in tables)
- transforming data into a common rubric (name of a particular group or section), for example changing actual numbers from different papers into percentages
- charts, which can include histograms, pie charts and other types
- translating data either by a thematic or content analysis.

> ### Practical Tip
>
> We recommend that prior to commencing the systematic review you look at the various tools and checklists available to find one that best suits you and your review.

How and where to get started on presenting your results

This section discusses how to go about summarizing, synthesizing and presenting your results. There are a number of different ways you can do this. The methods for summarizing and synthesizing your data discussed within this book are primarily aimed at the novice reviewer. For more experienced reviewers, the PRISMA (Preferred Reporting Items for Systematic Reviews and Meta-Analyses) document outlines how systematic reviews should be reported for academic journals. For more comprehensive information about PRISMA, see Equator Network (2024) and Page et al. (2021).

Essentially, the results of everything you have done so far need to be presented, including:

---

1. Presenting the results of your search
2. Presenting the results of the studies selected based on the title and abstract
3. Presenting the results of the studies selected based on reading the full paper
4. Presenting a summary of all your included studies
5. Presenting a summary of all the critiques of the included papers using the appropriate frameworks
6. Presenting a summary of the data extracted (including a synthesis of the overall results)

All the above will now be discussed in turn.

1. Presenting the results of your search

The results of the comprehensive search can be presented either textually or in a table. When writing the search up, it is important to identify all the databases that you have searched together with the results you found, so that anyone reading the review can ascertain how comprehensive, transparent and replicable your review is. When presenting the results, it is usual to include the databases searched with the dates included: the date of the search, the number of hits, the number of articles discarded as well as the number of articles left that need to be reviewed by title and abstract. Results presented in tables also need to be explained fully. Table 10.1 provides an example of how the results of your systematic literature review in nursing could be presented. *Please note that this is all fictitious information.*

Table 10.1 An example of one way of presenting the results of the systematic search

Database with dates	Search date	Number of hits retrieved from the search	Number of articles discarded because of irrelevant titles	Number of articles duplicated from another database	Number of articles to be reviewed by title and abstract
CINAHL (2000–2023)	20/11/23	1569	1456	79	34
MEDLINE (1963–2023)	21/11/23	1847	1346	244	284
EMBASE (1996–2023)	23/11/23	2485	1567	600	318

Practice session 10.1

For your own systematic review question, using the template (Box 10.1), try to fill in the databases you used when searching for your own systematic review question. Write down the dates included, the date of the search, the number of hits, the number of articles discarded and the number of articles remaining that need to be reviewed by title and abstract. As mentioned in Chapter 6 you can now see how important it is to document all your searches as you go along. If you don't do this, it will mean that you will need to conduct the search again.

Box 10.1 Template to use for presenting the results of your systematic search

Database with dates	Search date	Number of hits retrieved from search	Number of articles discarded due to irrelevant titles	Number of articles duplicated from another database	Number of articles to be reviewed by title and abstract
CINAHL					
MEDLINE					
EMBASE					
COCHRANE					
AMED					

2. Presenting the results of the studies selected based on the title and abstract

Once the search of a systematic review is conducted, the second step of the review is the selection of the primary research studies that meet your inclusion criteria, based on reading the abstracts and titles. Table 10.2 is an example of one way these results could be presented, based on the case study of Mary's systematic review on domestic violence. The first three columns have been filled in to illustrate this point. In column 1 the action is to include the paper, as all the criteria have been met. In column 2 the action is to exclude the paper, as two of the criteria have not been met. In column 3 the action is to read the full paper before deciding whether to include or exclude the study, as it is unclear from reading the abstract whether or not advocacy was included in the primary paper under consideration.

Ⓜ **Table 10.2** An example of one way of presenting the results of Mary's included studies based on reading the title and abstract

Abstract number	1	2	3	4	5
Population					
Women?	√	√	√		
Over 18?					
Intervention					
Advocacy	√	√	?		
Comparative group					
Peer groups or general practice treatment?	√	×	√		
Outcomes					
Women's experiences of interventions?	√	×	√		
Type of study					
Phenomenological	√	√	√		
*Action	Include	Exclude	Read full article		

*Include (read full article); exclude; read full article.

3. Presenting the results of the studies selected based on reading the full paper

The third step involves presenting the results of the studies included based on reading the full paper, and this can be presented in a similar format. The final action in this stage is to include or exclude the paper only. Presenting a table similar to Table 10.2 will enable you to know precisely on which selection criteria you have based your decision to select your papers. It makes the process of how you conducted your systematic review very clear, transparent and replicable. Remember to include the bibliographic details of the full articles (i.e. the names of the authors, the titles of the articles and the journals they were published in along with the country of origin) so the reader can know exactly which papers were included, which were excluded and why.

Practice session 10.2

Now use one of the templates provided below to present the inclusion results of the criteria you used for your systematic review. You should already have done this in Chapter 5. Please note that for the first phase of the selection of studies, your actions can be to include, exclude or read the full paper and then make a decision (Box 10.2). For the second phase where you read the full paper, your decision can only be to include or exclude (Box 10.3). Whatever type of systematic review question you have (i.e. either PICOT or PEOT), the results of the two stages you undertook to select your papers need to be presented.

Box 10.2   Template for you to use for presenting the results of the included studies based on reading the title and abstract and using the PICOT format

Abstract number	1	2	3	4	5
Population					
Intervention					
Comparative group					
Outcomes					
Type of study					

*Action: Include, exclude or read full article

Box 10.3   Template for you to use for presenting the results of the included studies based on reading the full paper and using the PEOT format

Paper number	1	2	3	4	5
Population					
Exposure					
Outcomes					
Type of study					

*Action: include or exclude

4. Presenting a summary of all your included studies

The fourth step is to provide a summary and present a description of all the primary studies you included within your systematic review. Ideally, the details of what is presented should be the same for each study. Tables 10.3 and 10.4 show two examples of how information could be presented in tabular format. In Table 10.3 the first row is filled in, as an example of the details that could be included for one study, using the case study of Mary's systematic review. In Table 10.4 you can see an example of what one of Sue's paper summaries on witnessed resuscitation could look like. In both versions, the information relating to all components of PICOT or PEOT need to be provided.

There is another way to present the details for all your included studies and that is simply to write a narrative summary with structured headings (similar to a structured abstract). If you choose to write it out this way, make sure that you include all the details relating to the type of research design, population, intervention or exposure and outcomes.

Ⓜ **Table 10.3** An example of how Mary could describe one study that she included in her review, based on all components of the PICOT structure

Study	Population	Intervention	Comparative intervention	Outcomes
1. Jones, M. and Smith, L. (2006) Effect of advocacy compared to usual care on women's quality of life. *Clinical Nursing* 20 (1): 56–60	Sample selection: Volunteers recruited from advertisements posted in various community agencies Number: 24 Mean age: 24 years old, range 21–51 years Abusive relationship status: 45% were currently in abusive relationships with no intention of leaving, 35% were trying to leave abusive relationships	60% are in individual counselling or a domestic violence support group	40% usual care	Quality of life (QOL) scales Advocacy group pre-intervention QOL values: 30/50 (50 is the average figure for QOL for healthy individuals) Post-intervention QOL values: QOL value 40/50 Usual care group pre-intervention: QOL value 29/50 Post-intervention usual care group: QOL value 30/50 (no difference in QOL post treatment)

Practice session 10.3

Select the appropriate template (Boxes 10.4 and 10.5) for your own systematic review question and try to fill in the details of your own included studies.

Table 10.4 An example of how Sue could describe one of her qualitative studies using the PEOT framework

Paper 2

Full bibliographic reference	O'Brien, J. and Fothergill-Bourbonnais, F. (2004) The experience of trauma resuscitation in the emergency department: Themes from seven patients. *Journal of Emergency Nursing* 30 (3): 216–224.
Type of study design	Phenomenological
Population	Four men and three women over the age of 18. Four patients were involved in motor vehicle collisions and three suffered falls.
Exposure	The lived experiences of patients undergoing resuscitation with and without family presence.
Outcome	To gain insight into the experiences of patients undergoing resuscitation as shaped by the context of their circumstances.
Results	Four main themes emerged: recollection, confidence in staff, lack of knowledge and experience of being a patient, and survival. These main themes consisted of numerous threads: frustration, feeling scared, pain free, kept patients well informed, lack of knowledge and experience of being a patient, tone of voice was calm and soothing, feeling safe, organized and caring, male patients thought family members got in the way, female patients felt that family members' presence was a source of comfort and reassurance, feeling important and comforted, going to get out, appreciation for life, positivity and vulnerability.

Box 10.4 Template to use for describing your included studies (PEOT format)

Study	Population	Exposure	Outcomes	Type of study
1				
2				
3				
4				
5				

Box 10.5   Template to use for describing your included studies (PICOT format)

Study	Population	Intervention	Comparative intervention	Outcomes	Type of study
1					
2					
3					
4					
5					

5. Presenting a summary of all the critiques of your included papers using the appropriate frameworks

In the fifth step, the summary of the results of your critiques can be presented in either tabular or narrative format. When presenting the results of your critiques, it is worth critiquing each study individually using one of the available critiquing frameworks or checklists, such as the Critical Appraisal Skills Programme (CASP, available at https://casp-uk.net/casp-tools-checklists/), Caldwell et al.'s (2011) framework, the McMaster framework, and so forth. You can then present a shortened version of the answers to all the critique questions for all the studies you included in one comprehensive table. This will likely run into a number of pages. Presenting the overall results of all your critiques in this way shows that you have appropriately and methodically critiqued the research papers that you have included within your review. Presenting the results of your critiques in this way is helpful when you come to discuss your review (see Chapter 11). Table 10.5 shows a hypothetical example for answering the first five questions for a paper using Caldwell et al.'s (2011) critical appraisal framework. Presenting the results in this way is helpful when discussing your results later in your review.

Although some critical appraisal frameworks, for example Caldwell et al.'s (2011) and the McMaster framework, do not yield a numerical value for the quality of the paper, for the purposes of your own systematic review it is still possible to assign values either for the overall paper quality or for each appraisal question based on your subjective appraisal. A Likert scale can be created representing the values of 1 to 5, with 1 representing a paper of very poor overall quality and 5 representing a paper of very good overall quality. Alternatively, it is possible to assign a numerical value to each question and then to add up all the individual scores.

The Caldwell framework has 18 questions. For each question you could have three possible answers (numbers) with an answer of no = 0 = not addressed, partly addressed = 1 and yes = 2 = fully addressed. The maximum value that any study could get using the Caldwell framework is 36. At this stage, if you plan to include only studies of good or very good quality within your systematic review, it is important that you state a cut-off point. For example, you could state that any studies achieving fewer than 20 points (out of a total of 36 points) will be excluded from your review. Alternatively, you could include all the studies (even the poor ones) and then conduct a separate analysis to assess whether the poor studies significantly affected the overall results of your review.

Table 10.5 An example of how to present the results for the full methodological quality (critical appraisal) of your included studies based on Caldwell et al.'s (2011) framework (first five questions only)

Paper	Q1 Does the title reflect the content?	Q2 Are the authors credible?	Q3 Does the abstract summarize the key components?	Q4 Is the rationale for undertaking the research clearly outlined?	Q5 Is the literature review comprehensive and up to date?
1	Yes, the title includes the research design, population, intervention, comparative intervention and outcomes. The title accurately reflects the content.	Yes, the authors appear credible. The first author has a doctorate in nursing, which shows her competence to conduct research. The other two authors are both registered nurses.	Yes, the abstract was very comprehensive and structured appropriately, with all sections included.	Yes, the rationale for conducting the study was very clear. The authors critiqued all the available literature in the area and very clearly showed the gap in knowledge, which they then proceeded to address.	Yes, comprehensive literature was provided. All the papers mentioned were also appropriately critiqued.

Practice session 10.4

For your own systematic review use one of the templates (Boxes 10.6 and 10.7), based on Caldwell et al.'s (2011) framework, to critique your papers. You may have already done this when you critiqued each paper individually, so it should now be a simple matter of cutting and pasting the answers from your individual critique to the template containing a summary of all your critiques. This will allow you to see the results of all the critiques you undertook in a collated format. If your original individual critiques are too long, you can cut and paste the most important and relevant information only. The two templates are similar. The main difference is that the template in Box 10.6 does not include a numerical value for each question, whereas the template in Box 10.7 does. If you decide to use Box 10.6, you can still rate the paper from 1 (very poor), which implies there was a high bias in the study, to 5 (very good), which indicates that there was low bias in the study, as discussed above.

Box 10.6   Template to use for presenting the summary of the results of the full methodological quality (critical appraisal) of your included studies based on Caldwell et al.'s (2011) framework (first five questions only)

Paper	Q1 Does the title reflect the content?	Q2 Are the authors credible?	Q3 Does the abstract summarize the key components?	Q4 Is the rationale for undertaking the research clearly outlined?	Q5 Is the literature review comprehensive and up to date?
1					
2					
3					
4					
5					

Box 10.7   Template to use for presenting the summary of the full methodological quality assessments of your included studies based on Caldwell et al.'s (2011) framework, including an overall numerical value

Questions for qualitative studies based on the Caldwell framework		Paper 1	Paper 2	Paper 3
1	Does the title reflect the content?			
2	Are the authors credible?			
	Background and literature review			
3	Does the abstract summarize the key components?			
4	Is the rationale for undertaking the research clearly outlined?			
5	Is the literature review comprehensive and up-to-date?			
6	Is the aim of the research clearly stated?			
7	Are all ethical issues identified and addressed?			
	Methods			
8	Is the methodology identified and justified?			
9	Are the philosophical background and study design identified and the rationale for choice of design evident?			
10	Are the major concepts identified?			
11	Is the context of the study outlined?			
12	Is selection of participants described and the sample method identified?			
13	Is the method of data collection auditable?			
	Data analysis			
14	Is the method of data analysis credible and confirmable?			
	Results			
15	Are the results presented in a way that is appropriate and clear?			
16	Are the results transferable?			
	Discussion			
17	Is the discussion comprehensive?			
	Conclusions and implications			
18	Is the conclusion comprehensive?			
	Numerical assessment awarded by author (maximum score is 36 points)		__/36	

6. Presenting a summary of the data extracted (including a synthesis of the overall results)

Whatever your systematic review question, in the final step the data you extracted will need to include details related to the study design, the population, interventions, comparative interventions (or exposures) and outcomes of all the primary studies you decided to include within your review. All these will now be discussed in turn.

Extracting data relevant to your population group

The way that data extracted from your studies are synthesized and presented depends on the type of data being handled. If you have quantitative data, the usual method is to present them either in tabular format or as a chart. If you have qualitative data, it is usual to present them in themes and subthemes in a similar way to how the results of a primary qualitative study are presented. With regard to presenting the details related to population groups, ethnicities and so forth, these data are usually numerical. For example, you might say paper 1 had 20 subjects, paper 2 had 40 subjects and so on. If you decide to include the religious affiliation of the populations you are looking at, you may want to consider using something like a pie chart or histogram. Table 10.6, Figure 10.1 and Figure 10.2 are examples of how you could present the number of subjects in each study. Charts and tables can be used to synthesize and present the population numbers in both qualitative and quantitative reviews.

Table 10.6 Example presentation of number of participants in all the primary studies included in your review

Article	Number of subjects
Jones (2010)	40
Davies (2020)	60
Smith (2021)	70
Bettany (2024)	80

Summarizing, synthesizing and presenting your interventions and comparative interventions

The types of interventions and comparative interventions used in all your included studies could also be combined to produce a pie chart or they could be presented in a table. Table 10.7 illustrates how the percentages of participants in the intervention and control interventions could be presented. The pie chart (Figure 10.3) shows an alternative method that could be used.

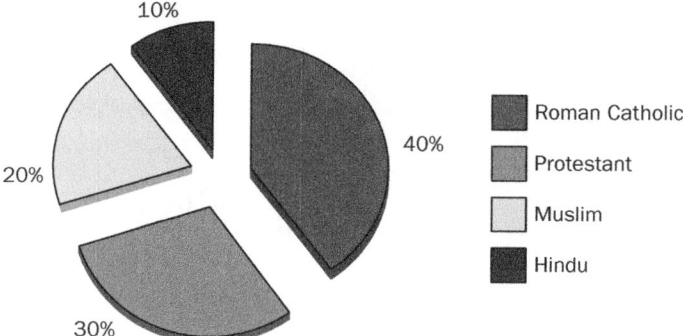

Figure 10.1 An example of how the religious affiliation for all subjects in all included studies could be presented.

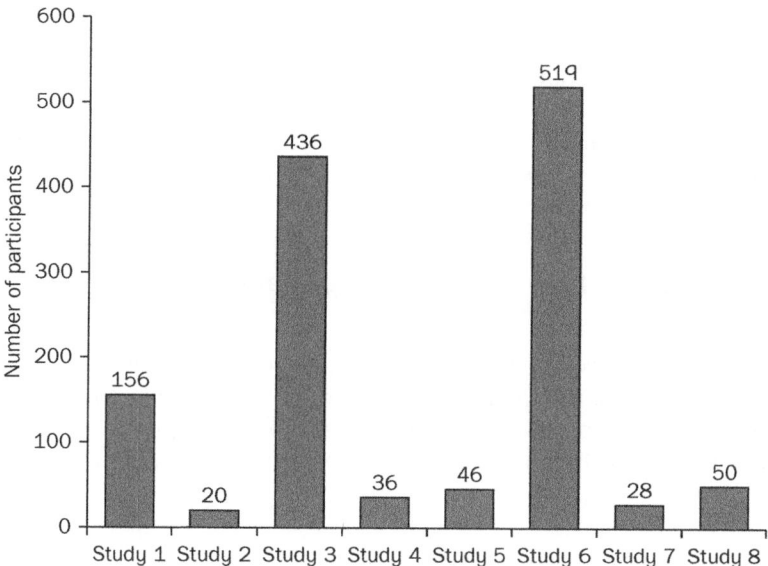

Figure 10.2 The number of subjects in all the included studies.

Table 10.7 Types of interventions in all included studies

Type of intervention	Number of subjects
Group advocacy	30%
Individual sessions	10%
Both	10%
Usual care	50%

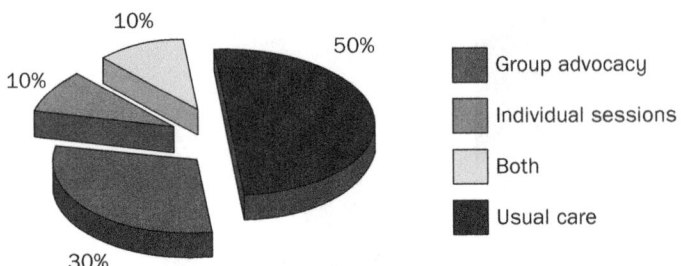

Figure 10.3 Number of subjects in each type of intervention from all included studies.

Summarizing, synthesizing and presenting your outcomes

The summary of the outcomes of the data extracted depends on the type of data you are handling. If you are synthesizing quantitative data, the usual method is to present the data either in tabular format or as a chart or other alternative graphical format. If the data you have extracted are qualitative data – that is, words – it is usually easier to present the data through the presentation of themes and subthemes. It is important when quoting anything to write down exactly where in the primary paper you got this information from (i.e. state the page, column and line numbers of the original primary paper) as you will be referring to this later when you discuss them within the discussion section of your review.

Summarizing, synthesizing and presenting quantitative outcome measures

Ⓜ Outcome measures provide the answer to the research question. As with the population and intervention, the QOL scores in Mary's case example could be presented in a table or a graph. Table 10.8 and Figure 10.4 show examples of how Mary could present the combined QOL scores from all her primary studies, both before and after the interventions.

Ⓜ **Table 10.8** Mean quality-of-life scores before and after advocacy intervention and usual care for all included studies

Mean quality of life scores for each article as measured by the SF-36 scale

	Advocacy group		Usual care group	
	Before	After	Before	After
Jones (2003)	30/50	40/50	29/50	30/50
Davies (2007)	25/50	38/50	24/50	26/50
Smith (1994)	23/50	41/50	23/50	24/50
Bettany (2008)	21/50	44/50	18/50	17/50

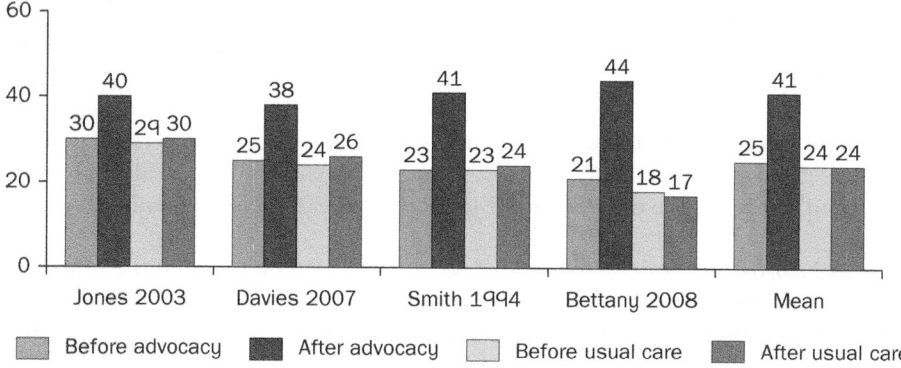

Figure 10.4 Mean quality-of-life scores before and after advocacy intervention compared to usual care for all included studies.

Summarizing, synthesizing and presenting qualitative outcome measures

§ As stated previously qualitative outcome measures are generally synthesized and presented under themes and subthemes in qualitative primary studies. Presenting qualitative outcomes in systematic literature reviews is no different. Sue could present the outcomes from her qualitative systematic review on witnessed resuscitation in various ways. Sue had three population groups: the patients, the families of the patients and healthcare professionals (HCPs). Sue's aim was to appraise their views and perspectives and compare any similarities and differences between them that would impact on or change nursing practice. Below are examples of how Sue could synthesize the outcomes from two of her population groups (the patients and the HCPs) under themes and present them in a clear format.

Sue found that three main themes emerged from the patients' experiences of resuscitation and invasive procedures, as follows:

- Theme 1: Recollection of the resuscitation and survival instinct
- Theme 2: Family presence
- Theme 3: Confidence in staff.

One way Sue could present the qualitative outcomes is presented below.

Theme 1: Recollection of the resuscitation and survival instinct. Seven out of ten studies included in this systematic literature review identified recollections of fear and frustration by the patient during the resuscitation event, which changed when they saw or heard the voice of a family member. Because of their family member's presence, the patient felt less alone, and more loved and supported. The extracts below illustrate this:

> I was very scared. I thought I would never have a leg again. I thought I might die. I remember waking up and seeing all those doctors. I was like, where am I?

> Something is wrong! I looked over and saw my dad and my mother. They were there to help me, to hold my hand, to give me a hug. (Eichhorn et al. 2001, page 51, col. 1, lines 22–28)

> It would have been awful to be there alone and have no family there by your side. I was scared that the lumbar puncture was going to hurt. I was afraid. Having him [my dad] there was so comforting. (Eichhorn et al. 2001, page 52, col. 1, lines 1–10)

Theme 2: Family presence. Five out of ten studies also highlighted the importance of family presence, which was a key motivational factor in the patients' belief that they would get out of the accident and emergency (A&E) department and return to pre-injury life:

> When I knew I was OK – and it's hard to tell why I knew it, but I knew the moment that they started coming around and checking me, I knew that I was going to be OK. I knew it with a surety, especially when I saw my mum and dad were beside me and would be there to help me recover. (O'Brien and Fothergill-Bourbonnais 2004, page 221, col. 2, lines 17–32)

Theme 3: Confidence in staff. Six out of ten papers showed that patients had great confidence (trust and faith) in the medical professionals. The extracts below highlight very clearly the strong support and admiration for the healthcare team when the patients sensed and received comfort from the staff and were kept well informed of the procedures that they (the patients) were undergoing:

> They warned me there was going to be lots of staff and not to be concerned . . . I felt they were treating me as if I were important. (O'Brien and Fothergill-Bourbonnais 2004, page 221, col. 1, lines 19–24)

> They always kept me informed . . . that's a very positive reassurance for me that I was part of the team getting me better. (O'Brien and Fothergill-Bourbonnais 2004, page 220, col. 2, lines 5–11)

For HCPs' experiences of resuscitation and/or invasive procedures, Sue could report the themes and extracts from her data extraction and synthesis of the professionals' perceptions as follows. Sue found that two main themes emerged from HCPs' experiences of resuscitation and invasive procedures:

- Theme 1: Judgement call
- Theme 2: Threat to comfort zone of HCPs.

Sue could illustrate these two themes in the following way.

Theme 1: Judgement call. All the primary qualitative papers identified issues relating to staff having to decide whether the situation was viable for family member presence:

> And what is more important, giving the person the right drug or trying to walk around family? I think space is the issue here. (Timmermans 1997, page 158, col. 1, lines 4–5)

The perceived lack of medical knowledge among the patient's family also contributed to HCPs' decisions as to whether to include or exclude the relatives, as can be seen from the following extract:

> As a layperson, I think it adds insult to injury because there are so many traumatic things that happen therapeutically from a medical perspective but could be perceived as additional trauma. (Knott and Kee 2005, page 195, col. 1, lines 30–45)

Theme 2: Threat to comfort zone of HCPs. Another theme which surfaced within all the papers was the challenge that family presence presented to HCPs during the resuscitation or invasive procedure. Family members being present within the resuscitation room made staff question their confidence in their own skills, thus contributing to stressful outcomes for staff as they attempted to do their jobs. This is clearly seen from the following two extracts:

> OK, let's face it, this is why it makes us uncomfortable. When we are doing resuscitations, we are off ... it is a mechanical thing. We don't want it to be just a mechanical thing, we want it to be a caring thing and yet we want to remain emotionally aloof so that we can feel that we can function better. We certainly don't want to ever make mistakes in front of a family member. You mix up the drug boxes sometimes. Sometimes you forget to take off a tourniquet ... Sometimes these things happen. You don't want to ever have a family see you make a mistake in resuscitation. For the family member that is just terrible. You don't want to have something go wrong – an IV gets pulled out accidentally. (Timmermans 1997, page 158, col. 1, lines 29–40)

> But you do feel like you're on stage, like somebody's watching your performance. But I'm pretty comfortable with my knowledge and skills, so it doesn't really bother me to have somebody there, I just have a heightened awareness ... You know, we have to show the family that we're doing absolutely everything that we can do, and you start to feel like you're not benefitting the patient, you're actually increasing their suffering. (Knott and Kee 2005, page 196, col. 2, lines 24–39)

Accompanying these thoughts, another excerpt highlighted concerns that as the HCPs were conducting their job in an effort to sustain life, they may have appeared insensitive in their manner while conducting the resuscitation; this is viewed as being cautious and reflecting on their practice in a judgemental manner, a manner that the relatives may see as not treating their loved one in a caring manner but treating them as if they were 'a person with a condition':

> 'With every patient you just log on, do your work and that's it. It's not Mr So-and-so. It is a patient, a person with an aortic aneurysm, it's a person with bilateral femoral fractures, it is not a patient with a name and that'. When discussing being

present during the resuscitation of their family member, the HCP [healthcare professional] answered negatively, '... you are going to be in the way because you are emotionally involved'. (Goodenough and Brysiewicz 2003, pages 60–61, cols 2, 1, lines 24–39 and 1–5)

The extracts from both the patients' perspectives and the HCPs' perspectives illustrate that some of their views are similar: both parties are aware of the patients' needs. However, a number of their perspectives differ significantly. Although the patients feel comforted by the presence of their family members, HCPs are not always comfortable with this and sometimes feel that the relatives get in the way. These similarities and contrasting views will provide very good material for Sue to consider in her discussion section.

Practice session 10.5

If your own systematic review question is qualitative, try writing out the main themes and selecting the most appropriate extracts from the data you extracted in Chapter 9. It is important to highlight the extracts that provide examples of the theme you are trying to illustrate.

Key points

- The synthesis is a summary of the current state of knowledge in relation to a particular review question.
- In a quantitative systematic review, if the results are similar enough it may be possible to conduct a statistical procedure, such as a meta-analysis, to combine the results (Chapter 13 provides more information).
- In a qualitative review, the combined results of all the included studies can be synthesized under major themes or subthemes. This is sometimes called a meta-synthesis or meta-ethnography.
- Irrespective of what type of data you have extracted, it is important to always undertake a narrative synthesis of the results of your findings to help you decide what other methods are appropriate.
- Narrative synthesis is a form of storytelling.
- Narrative synthesis may be used in a number of different ways, including:
  - before undertaking a specialist approach such as a statistical meta-analysis or meta-ethnography
  - instead of a specialist synthesis approach because the studies included are insufficiently similar
  - when the review question includes a wide range of different research designs, including qualitative and quantitative designs.

- The key points associated with the data extracted to some review questions can be summarized as follows:
  - Are the data sufficiently similar?
  - Are there caveats (explanations to prevent misinterpretation) that need to be acknowledged?
  - Are there any particular trends or themes?
  - Do the data seem to point in one direction or several?
- There are numerous tools that you can use to summarize, synthesize and present your data; some of the more common ones include:
  - textual descriptions
  - grouping of similar data
  - transforming data into a common rubric
  - charts
  - translating data by either a thematic or content analysis.
- The results of everything you did in your review needs to be presented:
  - The results of your search
  - The results of the studies you selected based on the title and abstract
  - The results of your included studies based on reading the full paper
  - A summary of all your included studies
  - A summary of all the papers you critiqued
  - A summary of the data extracted (including a synthesis of the overall results).

Summary

This chapter discussed the issues that you need to consider when summarizing, synthesizing and presenting the results of your quantitative or qualitative systematic review in nursing practice. In the first instance a narrative synthesis needs to be included for whatever type of data you have extracted. This can be done by using a number of different tools to summarize, organize and condense your data. Additionally, the results of all the methods you have undertaken within your systematic review need to be presented. A key point when summarizing, synthesizing and presenting your results is to make sure that you present everything in a clear, transparent and easy-to-understand format.

Question and Answer (Q&A)

(Q) Does it matter how you present your results?

(A) It is important to present your findings in ways that best represent the type of systematic review you have undertaken, for example figures, tables and charts for a quantitative review and narrative extracts for a qualitative review. All the findings need to be presented in a clear, comprehensive, accurate and transparent way. Remember: another colleague may wish to learn from your systematic review, making it essential for all steps to be easy to follow.

References

Caldwell, K., Henshaw, L. and Taylor, G. (2011) Developing a framework for critiquing health research: An early evaluation. *Nurse Education Today* 31 (8): e1–7.

CRD (Centre for Reviews and Dissemination) (2009) *Systematic Reviews: CRD's Guidance for Undertaking Reviews in Health Care.* Available at http://www.york.ac.uk/crd/guidance/ (accessed 12 January 2024).

Equator Network (2024) The PRISMA2020 statement: An updated guideline for reporting systematic reviews. Available at https://www.equator-network.org/reporting-guidelines/prisma (accessed 24 January 2024).

Kim, E.Y. and Chang, S.O. (2022) A meta-synthesis study of person-centered care experience from the perspective of nursing home residents. *International Journal of Environmental Research and Public Health* 14;19 (14): 8576.

Page, M.J., McKenzie, J.E., Bossuyt, P.M. et al. (2021) The PRISMA 2020 statement: An updated guideline for reporting systematic reviews. *Systematic Reviews* 10: Art. 89.

Popay, J., Roberts, H., Sowden, A. et al. (2006) *Guidance on the Conduct of Narrative Synthesis in Systematic Reviews*, Version 1. Lancaster: Lancaster University.

Tranvåg, O., Oddgeir, S. and McSherry, W. (2016) *Stories of Dignity within Healthcare: Research, Narratives and Theories.* Keswick: M&K Publishing.

University of Toledo (2024) Evidence synthesis: Getting started. Available at https://libguides.utoledo.edu/n7920/synthesis (accessed 24 January 2024).

11

Writing up your discussion and completing your systematic review

Overview

- Structuring the discussion of your systematic review
- Summarizing your findings in words and numbers
- Discussing all the results you presented in the previous section:
    - Discussing the search results
    - Discussing the results of the studies selected based on the title and abstract
    - Discussing the results of the included studies based on reading and reviewing the full papers
    - Discussing the studies included in your systematic review
    - Discussing the quality of your included studies in a synthesized format
    - Discussing the data extracted (including a synthesis of the overall results)
- Developing and/or discussing the theory on how the intervention or exposure works
- Comparing and contrasting the findings of your study
- Relating the findings back to the objectives set out and the initial area of interest
- Pointing to any methodological shortcomings
- Discussing the ethical aspects of the included studies
- Discussing the findings with respect to practice
- Revealing questions for future research on this topic
- Stating some overall conclusions about the study
- Writing up your systematic literature review
- Academic writing skills: tips on style, grammar and syntax

Structuring the discussion of your systematic review

Docherty and Smith (1999) state:

> Structure is the most difficult part of writing, no matter whether you are writing a novel, a play, a poem, a government report, or a scientific paper. If the structure is right then the rest can follow fairly easily, but no amount of clever language

can compensate for a weak structure. Structure is important so that readers don't become lost. They should know where they've come from, where they are, and where they are headed. A strong structure also allows readers to know where to look for particular information and makes it more likely that all important information will be included.

Docherty and Smith (1999) suggest that the structure for scientific papers should include a statement of the principal findings, a discussion of the strengths and weaknesses of the study and its strengths and weaknesses in relation to other studies. The meaning of the study findings, as well as implications for practice for clinicians and policymakers, need to be discussed. Finally, the discussion section should conclude by highlighting the importance of addressing unanswered questions and putting forward suggestions for future research. How can you apply these suggestions to writing up the discussion section of your own systematic literature review?

To recap, by now you should have reported the findings from your studies clearly and concisely in the results section. The next step is to fully discuss your findings (as described above). Early research (Docherty and Smith 1999) as well as more recent studies (Purssell and McCrae 2020; Khan and Zamora 2022), along with institutions specializing in systematic reviews (CRD 2009; Higgins et al. 2023), reaffirm the importance of starting your discussion section with a summary of your major findings.

This should be summarized in words, not repeating the figures from the previous section. Discuss your findings through comparing and contrasting your results, and then relate your discussion to the background literature. Ensure that you do not just repeat the results section. The easiest way to do this is to discuss each section in the order that you presented it in the results section. Depending on the type of review (qualitative or quantitative) the theoretical frameworks are usually discussed within the discussion section (mainly for quantitative reviews), but some authors choose to combine the two (i.e. writing up the results and discussion together in the same section; this is done more frequently for qualitative reviews). A summary of the key issues that could be included in the discussion section are listed below and then described in detail:

- Summarizing your findings in words
- Discussing all the results you presented in the previous section, in the same order that they were presented, including:
  - search results
  - results of the studies selected based on the title and abstract
  - results of the included studies based on reading the full paper
  - studies included in your review
  - quality of your included studies in a synthesized format
  - data extracted (including a synthesis of the overall results)
- Developing and/or discussing the theory or theories on how the intervention or exposure works
- Comparing and contrasting the findings of your study
- Relating the findings back to the objectives set out and the initial area of interest

- Pointing to any methodological shortcomings
- Discussing the ethical aspects of the included studies
- Discussing the findings with respect to practice
- Revealing questions for future research on this topic
- Stating some overall conclusions about the study.

Each of the points above will now be discussed using fictitious examples and extracts from the four case studies we have been discussing so far in this book. The references used in the case extracts are for illustrative purposes only and are not included in the reference list. A few extracts from the Cochrane Review that one of the authors participated in are also included (Romano et al. 2024). Please remember there are a number of ways to do this, each of which will include some or most of the points below. Your discussion needs to be clear, comprehensive and easy for the reader to follow.

Summarizing your findings in words

T It is a good idea to start writing your discussion section with a brief summary of the review findings. You could start by discussing the types of research designs that were included. For example, in her scoliosis study Tamara could say something like the following.

> In answer to the review question on the effectiveness of braces for adolescents with idiopathic scoliosis, this review found only six studies that met the strict inclusion criteria. Three of these were randomized controlled studies and three were cohort studies.

Next Tamara could describe the three randomized controlled trials (RCTs) in more detail and briefly remind the reader about the results of these studies:

> One RCT (Beaver et al. 2009) compared rigid braces to elastic braces and found low-quality evidence in favour of rigid braces. The two RCTs by Smith et al. (2004) and Thompson et al. (2006) found low-quality evidence for the effectiveness of a hard brace versus observation alone. Unfortunately these trials looked at different outcomes and could not therefore be combined statistically using a meta-analysis, so the results were synthesized narratively.

Tamara could also discuss any issues that would allow readers to decide if the results were both applicable and relevant to their own practice:

> The studies included only girls, were all written in English and included only the angle of curvature in the frontal plane as an outcome. None of the studies looked at outcomes that were important to the patient, such as disability, back pain, quality of life (QOL) and psychological factors.

In other words, if the readers of Tamara's systematic review were nurse practitioners living in, say, Russia who had mainly male patients whose main problems were increased pain and a poor QOL, they would realize that these results would not be applicable to their practice. Tamara could also qualify her findings by stating that as there were only a small number of studies, the results need to be interpreted with caution.

Discussing all the results you presented in the previous section

All the results presented in the previous section should be discussed in the same order in which they were presented there.

Discussing the search results

The search results are usually discussed only briefly. You will already have presented details of your comprehensive search in the results section, so there is no need to repeat that.

> **Practical Tip**
>
> What is most important when discussing this section is to highlight any issues with the search process that may have adversely affected your search and produced biased results.

For example, did you search only English-language journals? Was your search truly comprehensive? Did you include hand searching of all relevant literature as well as a thorough search for all the grey literature (PhD theses, conference proceedings) relevant to the review question? Did you contact any key people in the field to find out whether or not they had further publications in the field? In summary, this is where you highlight what you have or have not done and how this may have introduced any bias in the results of your search.

T Tamara could say something like the following:

A comprehensive search was conducted to retrieve papers that would answer the review question. Reading the titles and abstracts of 90 papers resulted in only 20 papers that met the strict inclusion criteria being found. Five papers were then excluded after having read the full papers for the following reasons ...
[here Tamara would state what the reasons were]

A search for papers that were not available electronically was undertaken, as well as a search for conference abstracts and PhD dissertations that were available in electronic format. Key people in the field of scoliosis were emailed to ask if they had any unpublished literature that could be included in the review. No documents were found. A factor that could have caused bias in paper selection was that the search was restricted to English-language papers and so will have excluded any primary papers in other languages.

Discussing the results of the studies selected based on the title and abstract and the results of the included studies based on reading the full paper

The subject of this section should only be briefly discussed. Again, any key issues should be highlighted. If you selected only three or four papers out of a total of 50 or more original papers, it is necessary to provide a rationale for this. Maybe your inclusion criteria were too rigid, or perhaps you decided to select a group of participants on which not much had been published. It is important to discuss the papers that were excluded and the reasons for this in more detail so that the reader can understand why you excluded any potentially relevant papers.

Discussing the studies included in your review

In this section you need to provide a discussion of the common (or uncommon) features of all the studies that you included. The easiest way to do this is to go through the summary or description tables of your included studies and then proceed to discuss each part of the PICOT (population, intervention, comparative intervention, outcomes and types of studies) or PEOT (population, exposure, outcomes and types of studies) components individually. For example:

- If you considered the population group of all your included studies, you could discuss how many patients in all were included within the review: were they small or large samples? If the total populations of all your included studies amounted to a very small number, can you really generalize your results?

- How old were the participants? Did some studies have much older patients whereas others included only very young ones? Could these factors have had an adverse impact on the outcomes of your results?

- Were all the studies included conducted within the same type of healthcare setting? If some studies were conducted in a tertiary care setting and others were conducted in care homes, this would make the reader aware that the settings were quite diverse.

- Were all the interventions and comparative interventions exactly the same? If not, how did they differ?

- Were the outcomes evaluated in all your included studies the same? If not, how did this impact your ability to synthesize the results?

All the above are examples of questions that could be discussed depending on your specific review question. Here is an extract from Sue's case study on witnessed resuscitation:

> § The seven qualitative studies included within this systematic literature review utilized either grounded theory or descriptive phenomenology. These were chosen for this review as they focused on the lived experiences of individuals, aiming to gain an in-depth picture of the populations' feelings and perceptions of the phenomena (Holloway and Wheeler 1996: 15). Qualitative research is

beneficial to this review and healthcare research because it adopts a holistic (person-centred) approach. A person-centred approach is associated with gaining the overall picture of the life context, beliefs and values in the human environment. It is this aspect of the research that becomes a strength of qualitative studies, whereby quantitative methods would be inappropriate as they do not study subjective, humanistic lifestyles (Leininger 1985: 23). As identified by Holloway and Wheeler (2002: 6), quantitative research is useful, although it neglects participants' perspectives within the context of their environment. All the included studies were conducted in a similar setting, although the hospitals varied in whether or not they used protocols for witnessed resuscitation. Four out of seven of the studies included the perspectives of the patients and six out of seven the perspectives of the patient, the family and the healthcare professionals (HCPs).

In Sue's extract, she first provides a rationale for using qualitative research and why this specific methodology is the most appropriate for her review question. Sue clarifies the strengths of qualitative research for evaluating witnessed resuscitation and also explains why quantitative research would not be a suitable methodology. She then goes on to discuss her included papers in more detail.

Discussing the quality of your included studies in a synthesized format

Discussing the quality of your studies is one of the most important aspects of the discussion section and, depending on whether you are planning to write up your results as a report, dissertation or paper, can run into many pages.

§ In Sue's review, this section will be based on the individual quality appraisals that Sue conducted on each of her studies and which she evaluated earlier on, while conducting her systematic literature review. The key point that Sue needs to remember when writing this section is that the results of all the appraisals of the studies need to be synthesized or combined together to give the reader an *overall summary* of the quality of the papers that were included in the review. This part of the discussion will most likely be one of the longest subsections in the discussion.

You will also need to consider whether or not the quality of the included studies affects the outcome of your results. If the methods of a particular study or the study were classed as 'very poor', can you still believe the results and apply them to practice? Obviously you cannot.

Here is an extract from Sue's systematic literature review on witnessed resuscitation:

All papers addressed how the studies ensured trustworthiness. Credibility was highlighted in papers by Warren et al. (2006) and Crosby (2009) by utilizing member checking, whereby the researcher returned to the participants to achieve feedback on interpretation (Polit and Beck 2004: 432). This is considered the most important technique for establishing credibility, according to Lincoln and Guba (1985). Peer debriefing was also carried out in the papers by Andrews et al. (2005), Willowby et al. (2004) and Bell et al. (2010), as the researchers involved peers in reviewing different aspects of the inquiry. Data, investigator, theoretical and methodological triangulation was evident in some of the studies, which strengthens credibility.

Discussing the data extracted (including a synthesis of the overall results)

The data extracted included aspects relating to the PICOT elements for quantitative studies and the PEOT elements for qualitative studies. Once you have synthesized the extracted data, it is important to discuss this data in the discussion section.

§ Below is an extract from the discussion section pertaining to one qualitative outcome from Sue's review, which she discusses under a specific theme.

Theme 1: Threat to comfort zone and judgement call

Within this theme, several threads emerged relating to feelings among HCPs that family presence put additional strain on the team conducting the resuscitation process. This theme outlines some choices they had to make when deciding whether the family members should be present, depending on the individuals' coping ability. This view was supported by a patient in the study conducted by Eichhorn et al. (2001: 53), who was asked his opinion on how family presence could affect the healthcare environment. He disclosed that it was important that family members understand that they should conduct themselves in an appropriate manner and stated: 'It should be decided on a case-by-case basis – who can handle it and who cannot!' Knott and Kee (2005: 198) concede that they do not facilitate family presence for several reasons: (a) lack of space, (b) insufficient staff, and (c) the potential that the above may have to create psychological problems for the family member.

Here is an extract concerning the QOL outcome from a Cochrane review on braces:

Quality of life

Both rigid and elastic braces caused problems, though different kinds of problems. Whilst the rigid brace caused significantly more problems with heat (85% versus 27%), as well as difficulties with donning and doffing, the patients using the elastic braces had difficulties with toileting (Wong 2008). There is low quality evidence from one RCT (N = 43) that a rigid brace is hotter and more difficult to put on and take off than an elastic one, but an elastic one is difficult to maneuver during toileting. (Negrini et al. 2010: 1687)

In both the witnessed resuscitation extract as well as the brace extract, the key issue to be discussed is stated in the first sentence of the paragraph and then the rest of the paragraph goes on to explain what was stated in the first sentence. Thus, the first sentence sets the scene for the rest of the paragraph.

Developing and/or discussing the theory on how the intervention or exposure works

In this section it would be helpful, especially if the results of your review are positive or really important (such as witnessed resuscitation), to discuss the theories on how this intervention may work or how policies governing the intervention protocols could be improved or standardized.

T In Tamara's review, she could discuss different people's theories as to how hard braces and soft braces work, and what factors may influence whether they work or not, for example compliance (whether or not the patient wears the brace or not).

S Sue's review on witnessed resuscitation could discuss the importance of witnessed resuscitation to the patients themselves as well as the family, even though the healthcare staff may find it hinders them to have the family around.

Comparing and contrasting the findings of your study

Comparing your findings with the findings of other reviewers is also very important. This places the results of your review within the context of other research and reviews that have already been carried out. Do your review results support the work of others? Do they contradict them? And, if so, why do you believe this is?

T In the case of the scoliosis brace review, Tamara could compare her results with other narrative and systematic reviews and discuss the similarities and differences in the population groups, interventions and outcomes, as well as any methodological problems of the included studies. She could suggest explanations for possible similarities and differences. Below is an extract from the Cochrane brace review that one of the authors participated in (and on which the example of Tamara's review is based), explaining how this review was similar to and/or different from other reviews. Suggestions and explanations for this are discussed:

> An 'evidence-based review' (Dolan 2007) looked at totally different outcomes from those considered here: the 'rate of surgery' (failure of treatment) in braced groups ranged between 1.4% and 41%. This paper was based on retrospective comparative studies, and on retrospective and prospective case series results, all of which were excluded from the current review. Furthermore, only papers in English were considered, while those adding exercises to bracing were excluded. It was not possible to obtain a good uniformity of methods and outcomes among the papers [...] These problems could be overcome following the SRS [Scoliosis Research Society] criteria for bracing studies (Richards 2005). Moreover, excluding papers that add exercises to bracing should not be done in the future, because according to SOSORT [Society on Scoliosis Orthopaedic and Rehabilitation Treatment] criteria (Negrini 2009), this is a management criterion to increase compliance. In fact, papers including exercises [...] report very low surgery rates [...] comparable to the best results in the bracing papers reported above. (Negrini et al. 2010: 1689)

Relating the findings back to the objectives set out and the initial area of interest

Relating the findings back to the objectives is an important aspect of the discussion section, as the discussion is not a stand-alone part of the review. Here you need to relate what you found in your results back to your objectives and background section.

⚑ For example, Tamara could relate her findings back to her objectives as follows:

> The objective of this study was to evaluate the effectiveness of braces for adolescents with idiopathic scoliosis on curve magnitude. The results of this review suggest that there is low quality evidence for their effectiveness.

Pointing to any methodological shortcomings

Pointing to any methodological shortcomings or flaws in your systematic literature review, and how these may affect the interpretation of the results you have found, is one of the key aspects to include in your discussion. Recommendations on how these shortcomings may be rectified in future studies would also be beneficial. Addressing the limitations of the review enables your readers to judge what parts of the review you could have improved on. Knowing the limitations also allows readers to judge the validity of the results for themselves and how applicable the results may be to their own practice.

§ Here is an example of what Sue could have written for her review on this subject:

> § **Limitations of the systematic review**
> Due to the primary papers included within this review having numerous methodological shortcomings, the overall results of the outcomes were compromised. The process of reading the full-text papers to assess the methodological quality and the data extraction procedure was conducted alone (instead of in pairs), which could have given rise to bias.

Discussing the ethical aspects of the included studies

The discussion of the ethical issues within the primary papers that you included in your review is important. If you have evaluated papers that made no mention of any ethical approvals or informed consent of their patients, it is possible that the authors conducting the studies did not consider issues of informed consent, right to withdrawal and so forth.

§ As Sue highlights in her systematic literature review, ethical approval by local ethical committees is considered as an indicator of reliability and validity, since it ensures that the study complies with professional, ethical and scientific standards. Here is an example of an excellent discussion on the ethical issues within Sue's systematic literature review:

> § As noted by Parahoo (2006: 112), all research studies have individual ethical implications and these are sometimes more prominent in one design than another. Importantly, the process of interviewing vulnerable participants – such as those identified in this review – warrants serious ethical consideration. Papers 1, 4 and 5 clearly identify that either verbal or written consent was achieved from the participants and ethical approval obtained from either the Board of Managers in the

included hospitals or sponsoring University Review Board. Commendably, paper 4 identified 'beneficence' in providing a 'duty of care' as recommended by the Nursing and Midwifery Council (NMC 2004: 4). The studies all asserted autonomy and confidentiality by issuing a pseudonym to participants and identifying the risks against benefit of exposure prior to the study; they also gave participants the choice to withdraw from the study and access to transcripts. The latter is important in qualitative studies to validate interpretations (Van der Woning 1999: 188).

Discussing the findings with respect to practice

An 'implication for practice' subsection should be included within the discussion section. Improving and enhancing practice is one of the most important reasons for conducting your systematic review.

§ Here is an extract from Sue's review:

§ Due to the nature of this 'subjective phenomenon', unless one has been involved in witnessed resuscitation, it is difficult to understand personal choice. Although the studies delivered strong support for witnessed resuscitation, there were also concerns about negative issues. As recognized in the background literature and throughout this research, cultural diversity affects values, beliefs and behaviours relating to health and illness; therefore, responses will be subjective (Eichhorn et al. 2001: 54). Through awareness of our own capabilities, we as professional individuals can recognize personal perceptions and biases to accept family choice with respectful autonomy and provide a duty of care (NMC 2004: 4). Through conducting this systematic review it has been identified that further studies should be undertaken to gain knowledge from the patient perspective. One commonality between all the studies (except Paper 2) was the recommendation for a protocol to be developed to deal especially with the psychosocial requirements of relatives. In Paper 7, attitudes towards family presence changed from negative to positive. The paper advocated initiating a 'pilot' site in order to provide the necessary data to implement change. Change in this context refers to the introduction of protocols as well as education for HCPs and laypersons connected to family presence, on a national level in the UK (Hulme 2009).

Suggesting questions for future research on this topic

Suggesting areas for future research is a key aspect of any discussion. Include the main points investigated within your review that you would like the reader to remember, highlight what is still not known and include suggestions of the most relevant research that you think should be done to further improve practice in this area.

Stating some overall conclusions about the study

The conclusions of your review should provide a summary of the whole review and restate the key findings.

T An extract from Tamara's brace review is presented first. Her findings were very similar to those provided by Negrini et al.'s (2010) Cochrane review on braces:

Conclusion

Today the only alternative to bracing is the so-called 'wait and see' strategy (i.e. observation and eventual surgery). The scientific evidence is in favour of bracing, but quality is very low [...] any future study should look at patient outcomes (not just radiographic outcomes of scoliosis progression) as well as adverse effects, so that balanced conclusions may be generated (Negrini et al. 2010: 1689).

§ An extract from Sue's witnessed resuscitation review conclusion is provided next:

§ Conclusion

This systematic review has identified a plethora of views from patients, family members and HCPs surrounding their individual experiences of family presence during resuscitation and/or invasive procedures. Each group identified their preferences within themes that were explored through rich narration, thus giving an overall impression of trustworthiness, which will contribute to informing practice when utilized with expert clinical judgement.

Derogatory attitudes among family members and peers when identifying the research aims and objectives around the phenomenon of witnessed resuscitation are recalled by the author. This may be due to a lack of knowledge and understanding of the topic area and the complexities involved. On reflection, it would be interesting to find out their opinions of the topic after reading this review, for it is important that all individuals are given the choice to be present or not. We might experience being present during the birth of a loved one; therefore, could we not also be included in a loved one's departure from life?

The ability to understand this particular phenomenon can lead to nursing care that is responsive to the complex experiences of the life world in the resuscitation room. Supported by protocols such as those developed by the Emergency Nurses Association (ENA 2001: Appendix 4), practitioners can deliver truly holistic care. Until such time, family presence will continue to be highly debated until protocols are institutionalized to aid the decision-making process through relevant evidence-based care (Hulme 2009).

Writing up your systematic literature review

The final step in conducting your systematic literature review is writing it up to a high standard. Depending on why you are conducting your systematic literature review, you may need to write up a dissertation, a journal article, a hospital report or a paper for a commissioning body. Irrespective of where you are planning to write up your review, it is important to take as much care in writing it up as in conducting the review. The report should include all aspects of the systematic review process, including the background, objectives, inclusion and exclusion criteria, methods of selecting and appraising your papers, methods of extracting relevant data, the results section, the discussion and conclusions.

As discussed earlier, by the time you have written up the plan or protocol of your review, you should already have the first five major sections written up, albeit in the future tense.

Practical Tip

Once you have completed your review, having the protocol or plan written up makes completing the review much easier, as you will not be starting from scratch. In fact the first five sections or chapters of your systematic review should be mostly written up in the protocol (1. Background, 2. Selection criteria, 3. Objectives, 4. Search strategy and 5. Methods).

Once you have finished your review the aspects that you will need to concentrate on are the background section/chapter and making sure it is sufficiently in-depth. You will of course also need to write up and present all your results and discussion sections. You will also need to go back through your whole systematic review paper or thesis to make sure that you have appropriately and fully written up all the sections of your literature review. In Chapter 12 we have included a checklist to help you to do so.

Practical Tip

Another important point to consider are the tenses to use when you are writing both the protocol and the full literature review. When writing your protocol or plan you will need to use the future tense, as this is something you plan on doing in the very near future. However, when you complete you review it is crucial that you now change all the tenses to the past tense, as the review is now completed.

You will need to go back to your plan and update the background section (there may have been more papers or relevant reviews published by this time). You should already have your objectives, inclusion and exclusion criteria, methods for selecting and appraising your papers and methods for data extracting written up, although it will be worth checking them over to ensure you did what you said you would do in your original plan. You should now have only two major sections to write up – the results and the discussion sections, including the conclusion.

It is important to ensure that your report is written up clearly and with great attention to detail, similar to the writing up of a scientific paper. It needs to contain enough detail so other nurses or researchers can replicate your review just by reading through it. The literature suggests that poor-quality reporting of primary papers affects readers' ability to interpret the results. Many reports suggest that reviews (as well as intervention papers) often omit crucial details about the interventions or methods of the review, thereby limiting the ability of clinicians and readers of the systematic literature review to evaluate the findings. This also limits clinicians' ability to implement the findings in practice (Cochrane Nursing 2024). Ideally, similar to the writing up of your discussion section, it is best to structure the presentation of your review. Box 11.1 suggests how to present all the sections of the write-up of your report.

Academic writing skills: Tips on style, grammar and syntax

Many people assume that any literate person can write a research proposal and/ or a systematic review. This is not quite accurate. It is one thing to write a letter or an email to a friend when you go on holiday, but quite another matter to write in an academic style. You may want to consider finding and downloading an app onto your computer that checks your grammar, punctuation and syntax as you are writing. A further consideration is the management of all your references. Programs like Endnote or Refworks will help you manage all your references throughout the process of writing your systematic review. Moreover, once all your references are downloaded into Endnote or Refworks or similar you can instruct the program to produce your reference list automatically. This will save you a lot of time and effort.

Practical Tip

Writing is a complex skill to master and the only way that most people improve their writing skills is through practice, perseverance and dedication. Most students that we have supervised need to rewrite their paper or dissertation a number of times before it is of an acceptable quality for publication.

When writing up your report it is important to make sure you are using the correct tense. Before completing your report, try to check the spelling, grammar and syntax (this means the arrangement of words and phrases to create well-formed sentences). Reading a systematic literature review that is full of spelling errors is off-putting and gives the impression that the review was done carelessly and without attention to detail.

The following are some tips to help you write up your review and improve your academic writing:

- If you are stuck and have writer's block, try using mind-mapping exercises or brainstorming with colleagues.
- If possible, try to structure your work in advance.
- Know what you want to convey before trying to write it.
- Every sentence should contain one idea only.
- Each sentence should follow logically from the one before. A well-written text is a chain of ideas.
- When you write a new paragraph, introduce the main idea of the paragraph in the first sentence and then elaborate and give related examples in the rest of the paragraph.
- Try to link your paragraphs so that the text reads logically. If you put 10 different ideas in 10 different paragraphs and do not connect them in any way, the reader may think you are talking about many disconnected ideas.
- You could try to link the paragraph above to the one below by writing something related to the next paragraph in the last sentence of the paragraph before.
- While writing, keep your reader's needs in mind. This means providing a verbal 'map' of your document so that your reader knows what to expect, and placing verbal 'signposts' in your text to explain what is coming next.

Box 11.1 Suggested structure of a systematic literature review

Title

Acknowledgements

Abstract

Contents page

Abbreviations or glossary (if relevant)

Structured abstract

- Background
- Objectives
- Search strategy
- Study selection
- Study appraisal
- Data extraction and synthesis
- Results
- Discussion
- Conclusions

Main text

1 Background

2 Review question(s)

3 Objectives

4 Search strategy

5 Study selection

6 Study appraisal

7 Data extraction and synthesis

8 Results

9 Discussion

10 References

11 Conclusions

12 Appendices

Key points

- It is important to plan and structure the discussion section of your review.
- Start your discussion with a summary of your findings in words.
- Ensure that you discuss all the results you presented in the results section:
  - Discuss the results of the studies you selected based on the title and abstract and based on reading the full paper.
  - Discuss your included studies in terms of PICOT or PEOT.
  - Discuss the quality of your included studies in a synthesized format.
  - Provide a detailed discussion of the data extracted.
- Develop and/or discuss any theory or theories as to how the intervention (or exposure) works.
- Compare and contrast the findings of your study.
- Relate the findings back to the objectives set out and the initial area of interest.
- Make recommendations on how these shortcomings may be rectified in future.
- Discuss the findings with respect to practice and/or policy.
- Discuss the ethical aspects of the included studies.
- Reveal questions for future research on this topic.
- Finish your discussion by stating some overall conclusions about the study.
- Write up your systematic review to a high standard (this is a fundamental part of the systematic literature review process). Take as much care in writing up the review as in conducting the review.
- Ensure that you include all aspects of the systematic review process:
  - Background
  - Objectives
  - Inclusion and exclusion criteria
  - Methods of selecting your papers
  - Appraisal of your papers
  - Extraction of relevant data
  - Results section
  - Discussion section
  - Conclusions.
- Finally, take great care over the presentation of your review: check your spelling, grammar and syntax.

Summary

This chapter has discussed ways of structuring the discussion section of your systematic literature review. Extracts from case studies and a completed systematic review were presented. Suggestions for writing up your review report were described, together with tips for improving academic writing skills.

Question and Answer (Q&A)

(Q) What are the benefits of systematic reviews?

(A) There are several benefits in undertaking systematic reviews. They have the potential to inform policymakers, commissioners, regulators, professionals as well as the public with reliable sources of evidence. They support clinicians, academics and researchers in identifying gaps in the knowledge surrounding a particular area and/or specialty. They are effective in summarizing findings from the vast amounts of literature. They can help to improve safety, quality and care for patients, along with the culture and working environments for staff.

References

Cochrane Nursing (2024) About us. Available at https://nursing.cochrane.org/about-us (accessed 31 January 2024).

CRD (Centre for Reviews and Dissemination) (2009) *Systematic Reviews: CRD's Guidance for Undertaking Reviews in Health Care.* Available at http://www.york.ac.uk/crd/guidance/ (accessed 12 January 2024).

Docherty, M. and Smith, R. (1999) The case for structuring the discussion of scientific papers. *British Medical Journal* 318: 1224.

Higgins, J.P.T., Thomas, J., Chandler, J. et al. (eds) (2023) *Cochrane Handbook for Systematic Reviews of Interventions,* version 6.4 (updated August 2023). Available at www.training. cochrane.org/handbook (accessed 24 November 2023).

Khan, K.S. and Zamora, J. (2022) *Systematic Reviews to Support Evidence-Based Medicine: How to Appraise, Conduct and Publish Reviews,* 3rd edn. London: Royal Society of Medicine Press.

Negrini, S., Minozzi, S. Bettany-Saltikov, J. et al. (2010) Cochrane Review: Braces for idiopathic scoliosis in adolescents. *Evidence-Based Child Health* 5 (4): 1681–1720.

Purssell, E. and McCrae, N. (2020) *How to Perform a Systematic Literature Review: A Guide for Healthcare Researchers, Practitioners and Students.* Cham: Springer.

Romano, M., Minozzi, S., Bettany-Saltikov, J. et al. (2024) Therapeutic exercises for idiopathic scoliosis in adolescents. *Cochrane Database of Systematic Reviews* 2: Art. CD007837. DOI: 10.1002/14651858.CD007837.pub3.

12

Checking your systematic review is complete and a few practical ways to share and disseminate your findings

Overview

- Using the Preferred Reporting Items for Systematic Reviews and Meta-Analyses (PRISMA) checklist to ensure you have included all aspects of your systematic review
- Practical ways to help support you in sharing and disseminating your systematic review

It is important for you, as well as others who have conducted and completed a systematic review, to check that you have included all the necessary steps, information and sections deemed essential to producing a quality systematic review. This is regardless of whether you have completed this as part of a module, dissertation or thesis or if it is a separate piece of work or research. When we are teaching our undergraduate BSc and postgraduate MSc or doctorate students how to conduct a systematic review for their course, programme or independent research, we have found the PRISMA checklist useful. A number of other lecturers have also used this checklist to support the development of marking frameworks to aid the assessment process.

The systematic review checklist in Table 12.1 could also be used to check other systematic reviews, to assess whether or not the reviews have included all the relevant sections and addressed them appropriately. Another important aspect to consider when completing your systematic review is that of enhancing knowledge and knowledge transfer through sharing and dissemination. This chapter offers some practical ways to help support you in sharing and disseminating your systematic review results, be it at a conference, through a paper for publication or in the form of a report for your employer, funder and colleagues.

Preferred Reporting Items for Systematic Reviews and Meta-Analyses (PRISMA)

Before we go any further we would just like to say a word about the PRISMA statement that many of you may have heard about already. This statement was developed by a group of 29 review authors, methodologists, clinicians, medical editors and consumers. A Delphi consensus process was used to develop a checklist and a four-phase flow diagram (see Figure 12.1). The aim of the consensus was to agree on the items that most authors deemed were essential for the transparent reporting of a systematic

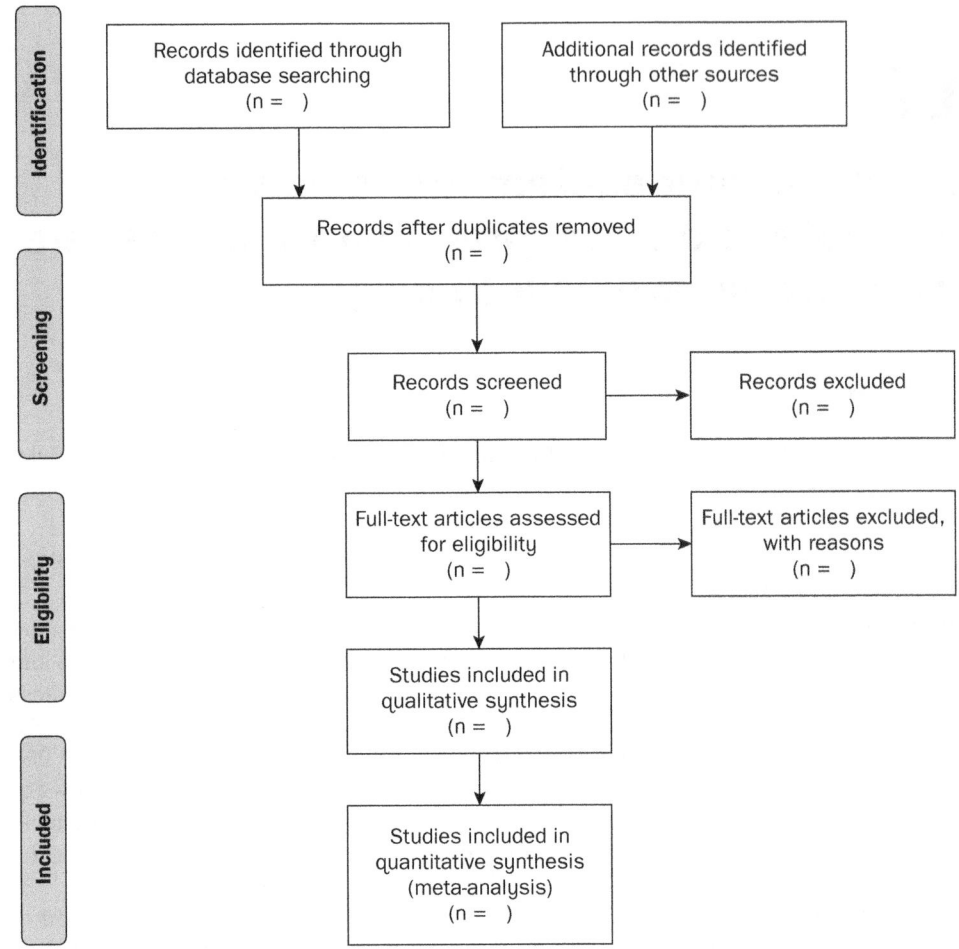

Figure 12.1 The 2009 PRISMA flow diagram.

Source: Moher D, Liberati A, Tetzlaff J, Altman DG,The PRISMA Group (2009). Preferred Reporting Items for Systematic Reviews and Meta-Analyses: The PRISMA Statement. *PLoS Med 6 (6)*: e1000097. https://doi.org/10.1371/journal.pmed100009. Reprinted under the terms of the Creative Commons Attribution License, https://creativecommons.org/licenses/by/4.0/.

review. After 11 revisions these authors approved the checklist, flow diagram and an explanatory paper that was published numerous times in different journals and websites to make sure it was disseminated as widely as possible (Moher et al. 2009).

You may find that a number of items on our checklist are similar to the ones included within the original PRISMA statement and subsequent updates. According to Page et al. (2021) the PRISMA statement was again reviewed and updated:

[To] ensure its currency and relevance, in 2017 an international group set out to update the PRISMA 2009 statement by incorporating advances in systematic review methodology and terminology occurring in the last decade. The PRISMA 2020 statement was published in March 2021.

A detailed description of the methods used to update the PRISMA statement is available in Page et al. (2021).

We have purposefully *not updated* our checklist, which was developed before the PRISMA statement was introduced. Our checklist is included as an aide-memoire to support you in checking that your systematic review is complete, with all the relevant sections included. We recommend that you use the latest updated PRISMA checklist, available at http://www.prisma-statement.org/.

We developed our checklist, shown in Table 12.1, primarily with the aim of helping you make sure that your systematic review is complete before handing it in for either your assignment or publication. It is worth noting that since the last edition of the book there have been many updates and adaptations of the PRISMA and associated checklists, which is why we have not included a new update of our checklist. By the time the third edition of the book is published there could be a new or revised version of PRISMA.

Systematic review checklist

The systematic review checklist provided in Table 12.1 offers an overview of what should be included within your systematic review. Completing the checklist should be undertaken to ensure that you have completed all the sections. You may also want to cross-check your checklist against the PRISMA statement/checklist.

Please note that not all parts of the checklist in Table 12.1 are complete. Our intention is to offer some illustrative examples. You may observe that some parts of the checklist are self-explanatory, which is why we have left them blank. Questions 1–5 have a column included to show if the required information was achieved. We would recommend that you develop your own checklist template for all the questions.

Practical Tip

If you read and review the systematic review checklist prior to commencing your review you will be more informed, confident and aware of the systems and process that are required in order to complete your own systematic literature review successfully.

Table 12.1 Systematic review (SR) checklist

Checklist question	Commentary/explanation	Possible responses
Title and question of the SR		
1 Is the title a true representation of the content?	Essentially what you are checking for is to see if the content of the SR is truly what the title says. For instance, having completed your SR, does the title include the words 'systematic review'? A good way to include this is to write your title as a statement, then put a colon and add 'systematic review' after this, for example: 'Comparison of surgical versus non-surgical interventions for adolescent patients with scoliosis: A systematic review'. Note: if you are writing an SR for Cochrane, however, it is slightly different, as they have their own format for writing the titles.	√
2 Has an appropriate question relevant to your area of expertise been developed?	Have you developed an appropriate research question and title for your SR? And is it within your or the authors' area of expertise?	√
3 Are all components of the question (PICOT or PEOT) included within the title?	Are all the PICOT or PEOT components written within the title and are these clear and easy to find?	? ?

If the SR is not your own, please check questions 4 and 5. If it is your own SR that you are checking please make sure that you are credible and have no conflicts of interest.

4 Are the authors credible? Do they appear to have the appropriate qualifications to write a SR in this area?	Do the authors appear to be appropriately qualified in this field from what you can read in the SR? The best way to check for this is to see what professions and qualifications the authors have by looking at the letters after their names as well as their place of work.	X
5 Is it clear from what you have read that the authors have no conflict of interest?	This is very important to check, because if the authors have a conflict of interest then there is a possibility that the results of the SR may be biased. So, for instance, if the authors were part of a company that made braces then their SR may be biased towards the effectiveness of this intervention.	√

Comments:

Abstract of the SR

6	Is there a clear summary of the research? This should include the background, objectives (and rationale), inclusion and exclusion criteria, search strategy, methods, results, conclusions and implications for the field. Abstract ideally to be no more than 350–500 words.	Here you just need to check whether all the sections are included and make sure to count the number of words in your abstract. This may vary depending on the actual criteria for your dissertation. Or, if you are submitting it to a journal, the word count may differ depending on the instructions to authors for that particular journal.
7	Is the abstract structured? If so, are all the sections included in the full SR represented and described in the abstract?	The abstract or summary of your SR needs to contain a description of each section of the full review. What we usually recommend to students conducting this type of dissertation is to write a structured abstract. What this means is that the abstract should contain the same subheadings as those contained within the full SR. In other words, the following subheadings: background, objectives (and rationale), inclusion and exclusion criteria, search strategy, methods, results, discussion and conclusions. This will make it easy for you not to leave anything out. What we have found over and over again is that if the abstract is not structured, students tend to leave one or more sections out.
8	If the abstract is unstructured, are all sections of the SR included and described?	If you need to go with an unstructured abstract then do make sure all the sections have been included. We have found from teaching hundreds of students to conduct SR dissertations that a common pitfall is to write an overview (in other words a more general abstract that does not give the specific details of each section that are actually needed).

(continued)

Table 12. 1 Continued

Chapter 1: Background

9	Is the introduction to the area well written and would it be considered capable of promoting interest?	In the introduction it is important to high-light the importance of the topic within the context in which it is used. As discussed in Chapter 4, you need to check that you have included statistics as well as key govern-ment documents to highlight how this topic or clinical condition is currently of great importance for patients and other readers.
10	Is there an explanation of how the review extends the existing literature? Or, if it is a duplication of another review, is it clear how your review is different?	For this section you are essentially checking how the review is extending what is already known. In other words, is this SR original? And if so, what other SRs have been con-ducted in a similar field and how is your review extending the current knowledge? Is it clear how your review differs to what is already out there?
11	Relevance of the study to the field or gap in knowledge, i.e. you need to show that no review exactly like yours has been carried out.	When you highlight the SRs that have already been conducted in this area it is crucial to highlight what these reviews have and have not addressed. The key point here is to very clearly show what is currently missing in these reviews; this should take you very nicely to clarifying the gap in the literature that your own review will address.
12	Does it demonstrate some knowledge of the special-ist area of practice? And does it question orthodox practice using balanced, logical and sup-ported argument? (This part needs to be contin-ued in much more depth in the discussion.)	Part of item 12 is generally addressed in the background section and then the rest of this discussion is addressed in the discus-sion section.
13	Are independence of thought and open-mindedness demonstrated?	It is very important to make sure that you are expressing your own opinions and crit-ical skills and not just taking all you have read in other papers at face value.

Comments:

Chapter 2: Objectives

14	Statement of the study's objective/s (or, if relevant, hypotheses).	As mentioned previously in this book it is important that the objectives are very similar or identical to the title. Do make sure that your objectives also include all the PICOT or PEOT elements (as the title also should).
15	Are the objectives (or research question) based on the background?	Do make sure that your title and the background are very closely linked.
16	Is it clear how these objectives will be measured?	Make sure that this is stated clearly, especially in the inclusion and exclusion criteria section.
17	Are they relevant to the clinical area under investigation?	Just a yes or no answer is required here, with the rationale.
18	Are they clear, concise and comprehensive, reflecting the title?	Just a yes or no answer is required, with the rationale.

Chapter 3: Criteria for considering studies in review

19	Have details of the types of participants to be included in the review been described?	In this section it is important to include who your population is, their clinical diagnosis, their gender, age range and time since diagnosis, together with your rationale – as well as who you will be excluding and why.
20	Have details been given of the types of intervention to be included in your review?	Make sure that in this section you have clearly stated and described the intervention/s that you have included in your SR.
21	Have details been given of the types of comparative groups to be included in the review?	Same as above, but for the comparative intervention. Tip: do make it very clear what the similarities and differences are between the intervention and comparative interventions.
22	Have details been given of the types of outcome measures to be included in the review?	It is important for you to specify precisely what outcome measures were included and how these were to be measured. This should include units of measurement, i.e. whether the outcomes in question are measured in degrees or centimetres, etc.

(continued)

Table 12. 1 Continued

23	Have details been given of the types of study (designs) to be included in the review?	Once again this is very important to specify. In this section you should have mentioned whether your SR only included randomized controlled trials (RCTs), controlled clinical trials (CCTs), cohort studies or just case studies (if for instance research in a particular field is very limited), or all quantitative or all qualitative studies etc. In the event that you are conducting a mixed SR then it would be appropriate to include both qualitative and quantitative designs.

Chapter 4: Search strategy

24	Have all databases that you searched been described?	When writing down the databases that you have searched, do make sure that you have described the name of the database together with the dates in years that it covers.
25	Was the search strategy based on components of the review question?	It is very important that within the search strategy section of your SR you describe **how you developed the search strategy from the actual research question**. Your search strategy should include *all components* of the SR question.
26	Were all possible sources of literature searched, e.g. electronic databases, MEDLINE, EMBASE, PsychLIT, CINAHL, etc.?	In order for your search strategy to be as clear, comprehensive and transparent as possible, all the databases, together with the years they cover, need to be listed. This includes the two sections below as well, checking specialist trial registers and hand searching.
27	Were specialist trial registers checked: Cochrane?	Yes, No, Unclear
28	Was hand searching undertaken?	Yes, No, Unclear
29	Were reference lists checked?	All references of all the papers you decided to include within the SR need to have been checked. Usually, many similar papers can be found in this way.

30	Was any grey literature checked, e.g. PhDs and BScs in libraries, conference proceedings or abstracts?	Do make sure you have remembered to include the grey literature. This includes, for example, PhD theses and conference abstracts that have not yet been published but that still need to be included in your SR.
31	Is the description of the search strategy detailed enough so that someone else could duplicate it and get the same results?	In the same way that a primary study needs to be able to be replicated, the search strategy needs to be listed and reported in such a way that a colleague of average intelligence could replicate it.
32	Were the numbers of papers located at each step of the search mentioned?	Many students and researchers use a flow chart to document each step of the search. If you look at most Cochrane reviews, they all include one. Please refer to Figure 12.1 to see what this looks like.
33	Overall, was the search efficient and used appropriately?	Here you need to check that the search terms and synonyms are actually derived from the research question and that the terms have been combined appropriately using Boolean terms AND and OR.
34	Have details of all three parts of the methods section been described?	For this item you just need to check that all three parts of the methods section (i.e. selecting, evaluating the quality of your papers or evaluating the risk of bias, data extracting) have been included.

Chapter 5 Methods

Stage 1: Study selection
The process of selecting papers for inclusion in the review (this process consists of two steps: the initial paper selection followed by the second, more thorough, selection of papers)

 Step 1 of study selection

35	Was the first selection of papers (for inclusion in review) based on titles and abstracts only?	This item is self-explanatory. When checking that you have both conducted and reported this, do make sure that it is clearly reported in your dissertation or paper. Ideally you should have included a subheading stating 'First selection of papers based on titles and abstracts'.

(continued)

Table 12. 1 Continued

36	Did you conduct it alone or did you and someone else perform it independently? If alone, did you state that this might affect (or have an impact) on both the reliability and the validity of the papers selected? (You may hear this referred to as selection bias in other papers or books.)	You will find that SRs conducted within Cochrane, the Campbell Collaboration or the Joanna Briggs Institute are conducted by more than one author. The authors will conduct the methods section (selection of papers, evaluation of methodological quality or bias) independently and then compare the results between them. This is done to increase the validity of these processes. If you are doing this SR for a dissertation, however, you will probably be conducting it on your own. This is fine too, but it is important that you have mentioned in your SR that because you have done the SR on your own the methods section may not be as reliable and valid.
37	Were the procedures to be used tested on a sample of articles (somewhat like a pilot study)?	Like in a primary study it is important to conduct a pilot study on a few of the papers using the standardized forms just to make sure that they work well and that you have included everything you need to select your papers and extract data from them.
38	Was a standardized form made for this procedure? Is it appropriate and adequate to answer the research question?	Here you need to check that the standardized form you created actually fully answers your research question.
39	Is a clear description provided of the criteria you were looking for at this stage?	For this item you need to check that all the inclusion and exclusion criteria for all aspects of PICOT or PEOT have been included in your SR.
40	Is it clear how disagreements were resolved?	For this item you need to check that you have stated how the two independent reviewers were selected and how they conducted the selection and review of the paper. If the two independent reviewers could not reach agreement on the review, then it should be made clear how an additional author was selected to conduct the review process.

41	Did you state how many papers were included initially and how many papers were left after the initial first selection?	Again please make sure that you have stated how many papers were included initially and how many papers were left after the initial first selection.
42	Are reasons provided for the papers that were discarded?	This item is self-explanatory.
43	Is it clear how disagreements were resolved?	This item is self-explanatory.

Step 2 of study selection (more thorough selection of papers)

| 44 | The criteria for this section are the same as above, except that the selection of papers is based on reading the whole paper. | This item is self-explanatory. |

Stage 2: The procedure for the assessment of methodological quality

| 45 | Was the appropriate checklist used to assess the methodological quality of each paper included in the study? For example if you used RCTs, CCTs and qualitative papers, then two checklists need to be included and described in this section. | As you may already know there are numerous checklists for various types of research designs. If you had a variety of research designs, it is important to check that that you have used the right checklist for that type of design. The framework by Caldwell et al. (2011) is easy, as you can use the same checklist to assess the quality of all your research papers. |
| 46 | Were the checklists or evaluation documents used appropriately and were they well cited and referenced? | Usually the documents for this item are placed in the appendix where your supervisor can check that you have filled in your checklists appropriately. It will ultimately help you to take some more time and use a book or explanatory guide to help you fill in the checklist items appropriately. |

(continued)

Table 12. 1 Continued

47	Was it clear how many people assessed the studies and how this was carried out?	The purpose of this item is to assess how valid your results are. Obviously if two independent assessments have been made by two students of the same papers the results will be more valid and less prone to error than if you conducted this process on your own. But, as we said previously, if you did conduct it on your own you need to mention it as a limitation of your study.
48	Were assessments done independently? If not, did you state the effect this might have on the results of the evaluation of the studies.	As above.
49	Was a description given of how the papers were evaluated? (e.g. poor, adequate, good, very good, excellent?) Or was a more objective numerical method used?	The Cochrane Collaboration does not actually use a numerical scale. They call the methodological evaluation the 'risk of bias', with greater risk being found in poor studies or studies lower down on the hierarchy of evidence. So RCTs will have a low risk of bias and a case study will have a high risk of bias.

Stage3: The data extraction strategy

50	Were the appropriate data extracted to enable the research question to be answered?	When checking this item it is important to make sure that you have extracted data for each part of the review question (i.e. PICOT or PEOT) and that these are clear and easy for a reader to understand and interpret.
51	Was the standardized form used to extract data appropriate to collect all the data necessary to answer the research question?	It is important to make sure you include all the data extraction forms in the appendix of your dissertation. If you are conducting the SR for publication in a paper then it is not necessary to show this work; however, we would suggest you keep the data extraction forms in case you need them while the paper is being reviewed.
52	Was the data extraction form piloted in any way before it was used in the study?	Again do make sure this is clearly mentioned in the appropriate section of your SR.

| 53 | Were data extracted by more than one student/ reviewer? | As explained above. |
| 54 | How were disagreements resolved? | As explained above. |

Chapter 6: Data synthesis (results)
Were all six sections of the results included (very important)?

55	Are the results of the search included and presented?	This item is self-explanatory. The results of your search can be presented either in a table or, better still, in the freely available template (Figure 12.1) available from the PRISMA website.
56	Are all the results of the studies selected based on the title and abstract clearly presented?	This item is self-explanatory. Please see Chapter 10 for a full explanation of this.
57	Are the results of the included studies based on reading the full paper presented?	Please see Chapter 10 for a full explanation of this.
58	Is a summary of all the included studies within your SR presented and were all PICOT parts included?	Please see Chapter 10 for a full explanation of this.
59	Is a summary of all the critiques of the papers using the appropriate frameworks included?	This item is self-explanatory. Please see Chapter 10 for a full explanation of this.
60	Is a summary of the data extracted presented (including a synthesis of the overall results)?	Please see Chapter 10 for a full explanation of this.
61	Are the results presented in an effective format?	Please see Chapter 10 for a full explanation of this.
62	Is the presentation of tables and/or figures clear and complete?	Please see Chapter 10 for a full explanation of this.
63	Has duplication of data presentation been avoided?	This item is self-explanatory. Please see Chapter 10 for a full explanation of this.

(continued)

Table 12. 1 Continued

64	Has text been used to clarify trends within the data?	This item is self-explanatory. Please see Chapter 10 for a full explanation of this.
65	Were the data appropriately synthesized?	This item is self-explanatory. Please see Chapter 10 for a full explanation of this.
66	Are the standardized forms on which all the data were collected included in the appendix? Were they appropriately filled in? (This item is for dissertations only.)	This item is self-explanatory.

Chapter 7: Discussion and conclusions

67	Have you demonstrated a comprehensive and detailed knowledge of the specialist area of practice and questioned orthodox practice using balanced, logical and supported argument (continued from background)?	This item is self-explanatory.
68	Is the interpretation of the results discussed with respect to theory, research literature, practice and ethics?	This item is self-explanatory.
69	Is the overall quality of the included studies discussed?	This item is self-explanatory.
70	Are the implications of the review discussed?	This item is self-explanatory.
71	Are the major deficiencies of the review discussed?	This item is self-explanatory.
72	Are the conclusions and the main relevant findings clearly summarized?	This item is self-explanatory.
73	Are recommendations made for future research and/or reviews?	This item is self-explanatory.

(continued)

References

74	Is the Harvard format used?	This item is self-explanatory.
75	Do citations and references match?	This item is self-explanatory.
76	Are the references accurately presented?	This item is self-explanatory.
77	Did you include a wide range and scope of papers?	This item is self-explanatory.

Presentation

78	Has the correct layout been used for title page, contents, page numbers, and so forth?	This item is self-explanatory.
79	Is the text free from errors and spelling mistakes?	This item is self-explanatory.
80	Is there appropriate use of vocabulary and grammar?	This item is self-explanatory.
81	Is there appropriate use of the appendices?	This item is self-explanatory.
82	Is there a logical and clear presentation of appendices?	This item is self-explanatory.
83	Is there a clear and aesthetic style and presentation of the report as a whole?	This item is self-explanatory.

Overall comments:

Key to possible responses on the systematic review checklist

√ This sign shows you have included the item and addressed it appropriately.

? This sign suggests that you are not sure whether you have or have not addressed the item correctly and/or in sufficient detail. You will need to go back to your paper/dissertation to check whether or not you have included it and sufficiently addressed this issue.

X This sign shows that you have not included this item or you have not addressed it correctly. You will need to go back to this item in your thesis or paper and amend your work.

We hope that this systematic review checklist will help you to cross-reference your own systematic review to make sure that you have included all the required aspects for submitting a quality systematic review. Once all the aspects are complete you may consider whether to share or publish your systematic review. From our experiences we find that many of our undergraduate and postgraduate students are satisfied with submitting their completed review only for their relevant degree. They prefer to leave things there, which is fine. The thought of doing any more work and/or publishing their work seems to be a bridge too far. For some of our students, confidence is often the issue and the thought of having your work marked and then possibly peer-reviewed is a daunting prospect, which we do acknowledge and appreciate.

We do, however, actively encourage our students to think about sharing and disseminating their work in order to improve practice. The next section offers some practical ways to help support you in sharing and disseminating your review should you decide to do this, once your systematic review is complete.

Practical ways to help support you in sharing and disseminating your systematic review

There are numerous articles and books offering sound information and advice about the opportunities and challenges associated with sharing and disseminating research findings and how this is important to ensure that we practise using an evidence base. The failure to share and disseminate the findings from research and/or systematic reviews could have an impact on:

- building a knowledge and evidence base for nursing and midwifery
- informing healthcare managers, leaders and policymakers
- establishing impact and outcomes of care
- offering equity through knowledge exchange and translation
- advancing innovation and change.

Lavis et al. (2005: 35) suggest 'that systematic reviews of research evidence constitute a more appropriate source of research evidence for decision-making than the latest or most heavily publicized research study'. This is because the dissemination of the results and findings from original research and systematic reviews can contribute to:

- adding new knowledge to the field
- evaluating specific nursing interventions and practices
- focusing on improving the quality of nursing and midwifery care and interventions and associated patient outcomes
- helping services to adopt and implement innovation
- supporting the practice of evidence-based nursing.

Despite all the evidence highlighting the importance of sharing and disseminating the findings from original research and systematic reviews to improve the quality of nursing care, interventions and outcomes, why do some researchers not publish their findings? Timmins (2015) offers some useful and practical guidance on why some nursing research does not find its way to improving practice and informing decision-making. A key statement from Timmins (2015: 34) is the following: 'research undertaken by nurses, or in the domain of nursing, is not likely to be used by others unless it is useful to nurses and support is provided for it to be implemented in practice'. Two important words from Timmins' statement stand out for us when focusing on the importance of sharing and disseminating findings from research: 'useful' and 'support'.

We believe that when focusing on sharing and disseminating the findings from research and or systematic reviews the researcher should think about the following. 'Sharing' is defined as 'to receive, use, in common with others' and 'dissemination' is 'to scatter far and wide' (Collins English Dictionary 1987). If you focus on sharing your work by making it 'useful', accessible and easy to read, and seek 'support' from supervisors, colleagues and journal editors to ensure your research findings are shared widely, we could see fruit in terms of further improvements in care and services. This is because nurses and midwives will be more comfortable about reading, reviewing and taking action on the findings and recommendations from your work.

The Centre for Reviews and Dissemination (CRD 2009: 85) defines dissemination as:

> A planned and active process that seeks to ensure that those who need to know about a piece of research get to know about it and can make sense of the findings. As such it involves more than making research accessible through traditional mediums of academic journals and conference presentation.

We would suggest that an effective strategy and action plan for sharing and disseminating your findings from a systematic review should focus on achieving the following:

- Ensuring that the essential message(s) from the findings reach the specific target audience(s) associated with the area of practice reviewed.
- Providing the findings in a format or style that is both accessible and relevant to frontline nurses and midwives.

Having identified a strategy and action plan for the sharing and dissemination of your findings it is important to identify some possible ways to publish your findings. Ohio State University (2024) offers some useful suggestions.

Practical Tip

If everyone who undertakes nursing research and a systematic review decides not to publish their work, how will the nursing profession continue to improve for the future? By publishing your work, you are contributing to furthering the profession.

We would suggest that to achieve evidence-based nursing, you need to be evidence-informed, which involves 'a highly complex series of systems and processes pertaining to how evidence is used to support decisions made in clinical practice' (Kumah et al. 2022: 328). To ensure that we are all evidence informed, the challenge for those who have undertaken a systematic review is in devising a strategy for the sharing and dissemination of your research findings. This is important in order to inform the evidence base of nursing.

🔑 Key points

- Once you have finished your review and/or dissertation, check that you have included all the steps essential to conducting a good systematic review.
- The systematic review checklist in this chapter offers a compressive overview of what should be included in your systematic review.
- The systematic review checklist provided in this chapter will enable you to cross-reference that you have included all the required aspects for your review.
- We would actively encourage you to think about sharing and disseminating your work in order to improve practice.
- Devising an effective strategy and action plan for the sharing and dissemination of your findings from your systematic review will aid you in publishing your review.

Summary

The chapter provided a detailed systematic review checklist and some practical advice and guidance on how and why it is important to consider sharing and disseminating the findings from your review.

Question and Answer (Q&A)

(Q) Who are the users of systematic reviews?

(A) The findings from a systematic review can be used by a variety and diversity of stakeholders. These include doctors, nurses, researchers, policymakers, patients, commissioners and insurers, to name but a few.

References

Caldwell, K., Henshaw, L. and Taylor, G. (2011) Developing a framework for critiquing health research: An early evaluation. *Nurse Education Today* 31 (8): e1–7.

CRD (Centre for Reviews and Dissemination) (2009) *Systematic Reviews: CRD's Guidance for Undertaking Reviews in Health Care*. Available at http://www.york.ac.uk/crd/guidance/ (accessed 26 April 2023).

Kumah, E.A., McSherry, R., Bettany-Saltikov, J. and Van Schaik, P. (2022) Evidence-informed practice: Simplifying and applying the concept for nursing students and academics. *British Journal of Nursing* 24;31 (6): 322–330.

Lavis, J., Davies, H., Oxman, A., Denis, J.L., Goldend-Biddle, K. and Ferlie, E. (2005) Towards systematic reviews that inform healthcare management and policy making. *Journal of Health Service Research and Policy* 1 (1): 35–48.

Moher, D., Liberati, A., Tetzlaff, J., Altman, D.G. and the PRISMA Group (2009) Preferred Reporting Items for Systematic reviews and Meta-Analyses: The PRISMA Statement. *British Medical Journal* 339: b2535. Available at https://www.bmj.com/content/339/bmj.b2535 (accessed 31 January 2021).

Ohio State University (2024) Health Science Library: Disseminate your report. Available at https://hslguides.osu.edu/systematic_reviews/disseminate#s-lg-box-18832635 (accessed 31 January 2024).

Page, M.J., McKenzie, J.E., Bossuyt, P.M. et al. (2021) The PRISMA 2020 statement: An updated guideline for reporting systematic reviews. *Systematic Reviews* 10: 89.

Timmins, F. (2015) Disseminating nursing research. *Nursing Standard* 29 (48): 34–39.

13

An introduction to meta-analysis

John Franklin

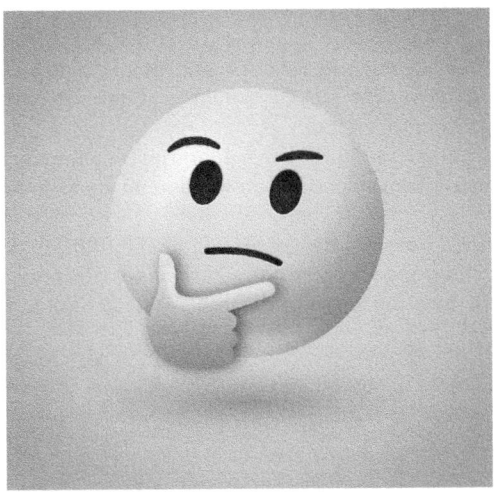

© Vilmos Varga/Shutterstock

When I was interviewed for my first fixed-term lecturing job, one of the professors asked me if I knew the difference between a systematic review and a meta-analysis. I won't lie – I didn't know! But I guessed that the framing of the question probably indicated that they were different. So, I went for it, and said I know they are different, I just can't tell you why they're different. To which there was some laughs in the room. Needless to say, I left the room and quickly googled the answer! And the answer is simple. A systematic review is a research methodology, and a meta-analysis is a data analysis approach.

Introducing the author

Dr John Franklin is a senior lecturer in Research Methods in the School of Health and Life Sciences at Teesside University in the northeast of England. John was mentored by Josette in how to conduct systematic reviews in 2009 and has been teaching students across healthcare programmes ever since. John's own research area, and the topic of his PhD, is chronic fatigue and he has a keen interest in research methodologies. John has helped develop over five hundred systematic review proposals at both undergraduate and postgraduate level and has published his own systematic reviews and meta-analyses.

Aim of this chapter

This chapter is designed as an entry-level introduction to the topic of meta-analysis, and I hope that over the course of this chapter I can introduce you to some of the key ideas involved and also help you develop your understanding. With this in mind, if you are planning on conducting a meta-analysis and writing this up for publication, I would recommend you seek support from an experienced systematic reviewer or statistician who can assist you in meeting the necessary benchmarks for publication.

Overview

- What is a meta-analysis? Why do a meta-analysis?
- Meta-analysis example and example forest plots
- Heterogeneity (or between study difference) and the statistics used to assess it
- Running a basic meta-analysis in SPSS (Statistical Package for the Social Sciences)

What is a meta-analysis?

In brief, a meta-analysis is a statistical analysis approach. You can have a systematic review without a meta-analysis, and you can conduct a meta-analysis on data that were collated without undertaking a rigorous systematic review. They are not synonymous terms; however, they are very much associated with each other.

Practical Tip

A meta-analysis is a data analysis technique. It is different to a systematic review. You can have a systematic review with or without a meta-analysis.

When are systematic reviews undertaken without a meta-analysis?

What's important to know is that systematic reviews are often undertaken with no meta-analysis included. To be honest this is usually because it would be inappropriate to do so in the first place. To run a meta-analysis the studies that you have included will need to have very similar PICOT/PEOT components. If the interventions are too dissimilar or the study designs are not the same, then you should not run a meta-analysis.

Practical Tip

We can only run a meta-analysis if the PICOT/PEOT components are the same or very similar – it would be inappropriate to use a meta-analysis if there is too much difference between the population, intervention and study type.

However, the good news is that there is guidance on what to do in this instance, such as the synthesis without meta-analysis (SWiM) guidelines (Campbell et al. 2020), which can help you with how to report your results. There are also other techniques that you could use, such as narrative synthesis (Popay et al. 2006) or thematic synthesis (Thomas and Harden 2008). However, for the purposes of this chapter we're going to focus on meta-analysis.

Why do a meta-analysis?

Now you might be thinking: 'Well, I know it is a data analysis approach, but I don't really get what it is.' Let's try and look at this in more detail. A meta-analysis allows us to take the results from the individual papers and pool these together in a way which generates a new overall pooled statistic (i.e. results from individual papers combined).

This is a fantastic statistical approach as it allows us to pool them in a way that means each individual study will have different weighting in our overall pooled results based on its sample size. So, papers with a larger sample size will have greater weight in our pooled results and papers with small sample sizes will have a smaller weight in our overall analysis. By pooling the individual papers together, it also means that we won't fall into the trap of counting p-values; instead, we can look at the overall pooled statistic.

This is what makes a meta-analysis so powerful: it allows us to take the individual results from a number of individual studies and pool these together to create a brand-new overall statistic for all of the individual papers combined. This means that instead of having to read the results of, say, 8 or 10 or 30 papers, we can simply look at the pooled statistic from a meta-analysis and this tells us what we need to know and it's all in one place.

Random- vs. fixed-effect meta-analysis

When we decide to conduct a meta-analysis one of the questions we should ask is whether we will be running a random-effects meta-analysis or fixed-effects meta-analysis. In essence, a fixed-effects meta-analysis is based on the idea that there is a 'true' effect that we can find in our analysis. For a random-effects meta-analysis, the assumption is that there are multiple 'true' effects that can vary from study to study.

As most of the work I'm involved with includes healthcare research I tend to use random-effect models. To keep things clear, I will just be focusing on random-effects meta-analysis in this chapter.

In summary

- A meta-analysis is a statistical analysis approach that allows us to pool the results from individual papers to create a new overall pooled statistic.
- Papers with a larger sample size will have greater weight in our analysis.
- Papers with small sample sizes will have a smaller weight in our overall analysis.
- Pooling the individual papers together means that we don't need to count significant and non-significant p-values.
- Instead, we get something better: we get an overall pooled statistic. That is, all the papers are combined to generate a new overall statistic for all the included papers together.

Meta-analysis example and example forest plot

When we run a meta-analysis we generate some statistics, such as our overall pooled result. But we also get a figure that displays our results as well. This figure is called a forest plot. Let's look at an example of an output from a meta-analysis. Figure 13.1 is the output from a Meta-Analysis created for this chapter. In this example I wanted to look at the effectiveness of a teaching intervention to improve student nurses' literature searching skills. The intervention is online learning only, and the comparison group is traditional onsite teaching.

All of the included papers were randomized controlled trials (RCTs) and for this example we've used 'post only data'. This means that we've only extracted the data at the post-test and ignored the baseline data. (I'll explain this more later on.)

So, if we think about what we are investigating here, we have two groups – an intervention group and a comparison group. Our participants have been randomly allocated to one of two groups. The intervention group has received online learning only and the comparison group has received onsite teaching only. For this study we measured 'searching skill' before they received any teaching (to control for different knowledge levels at the start of the study). We then measured 'searching skill' after the intervention had been delivered. We then want to see if 'searching skill' was better in one group compared to the other. In a nutshell, that's a standard RCT design.

Literature searching skill was measured using a continuous scale; the higher the score, in this example, the better someone is at literature searching. For this type of study, we will get a mean and a standard deviation (SD) for searching skill in both groups. What we are interested in is the difference between these two means. If the means are the same, then there is no difference between the two groups. If there is a difference between the means, then the intervention either improved or made their score worse depending on its direction. Table 13.1 provides an example of how this is calculated. We subtract the control mean from the intervention mean, and this provides us with the mean difference.

Table 13.1 Example of mean difference (arbitrary units)

Study	Intervention mean	Comparison mean	Mean difference
Bettany-Saltikov (2024)	25.6	22.6	3
McSherry and Bettany-Saltikov (2000)	22.6	25.6	–3

In summary, for this example we are looking at mean difference. That is the difference in the means between the intervention group and comparison group. If there is no difference between the means, then the groups are the same – the intervention had no effect on the outcome (in this example 'searching skill'). If there is a difference, then the outcome improved or worsened in one or both of the groups.

Interpreting a forest plot

When you first look at this output it might look a little scary, but it's quite straightforward when we start looking at the information that is being presented. When looking at the forest plot in Figure 13.1 from left to right:

1   The first column is called ID. This is straightforward enough: this is the name of each of the studies that we've included in our analysis.

2   There is then a second column called 'Mean difference'. In this analysis we are looking at how big the difference is between the two means. For instance, if you subtract the control group mean from the treatment group mean you will get the statistic that is presented here, which is the 'mean difference' column. This is simply the difference between the means in the two groups.

3   If there is a large difference between the means, then we could argue there is evidence that the experimental group performed better or worse depending on the direction of the difference.

4   The last column of note is the 'Weight' column. This tells us how much weight each individual study has in our meta-analysis, and you can see that studies with a larger sample size have more weighting and studies with smaller sample sizes have a smaller weighting in our analysis.

5   The other columns ('Lower' and 'Upper') provide the 95 per cent confidence interval (CI) for that study's mean difference, and the columns 'Treatment sample' and 'Control sample' are the sample sizes for the respective groups.

Remember: our meta-analysis does not just pool the data together; it *weights each study by sample size*. However, as this is a random-effects meta-analysis it actually gives a little more weight to smaller studies than you would see in a fixed-effects analysis.

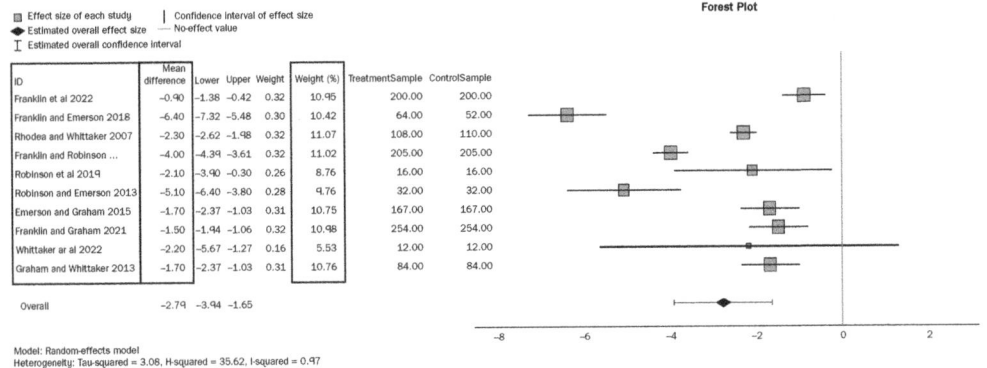

Figure 13.1 Example forest plot.

Now let's look at the forest plot itself. You can see on the image there are a number of squares and each of these are in line with a particular study. So, if you look at the first paper, the one by Franklin et al. (2022), you can see that the mean difference is –0.90 with a 95 per cent CI of –1.38 to –0.42. If you then move across to the image, you'll see that the square is at about –0.90. The square is showing us on the diagram where that mean difference is. The black line that goes through this is simply its 95 per cent CI. If the black line is short that means the 95 per cent CI is narrow; this is because the study has a larger sample size (and hence there is less uncertainty). However, if the sample size is small, then the 95 per cent CI is much larger (or the black line is longer).

Let's compare two studies in Figure 13.2. The top paper, by Franklin et al. (2022), has a total sample size of 400 and you can see the 95 per cent CI around this study's results is quite narrow. Now compare this with Whittaker et al. (2022): with only 24 people in this study we have a much wider 95 per cent CI.

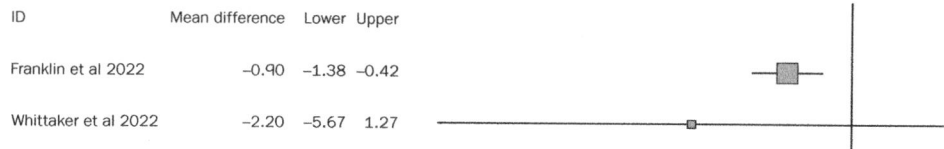

ID	Mean difference	Lower	Upper	
Franklin et al 2022	−0.90	−1.38	−0.42	
Whittaker et al 2022	−2.20	−5.67	1.27	

Figure 13.2 Comparison of two studies.

Nevertheless, all we have looked at so far is data that we have extracted and inputted into the analysis, just in two different formats: first the numerical data itself, second the data in picture format.

There are two other things that I would like to draw your attention to on the diagram in Figure 13.3. The first is the vertical black line at 0. This is the line of no effect and for a mean difference this is always 0. Something to note: if a 95 per cent CI of an included study crosses the line of no effect, then this study would have reported a non-significant p-value. So, on our forest plot all the included papers reported results where the outcome was higher in the comparison group. This is because when we have a minus value the mean in the intervention group must have been lower than the mean in the comparison group. Further still, 9 of the 10 papers reported statistically significant findings and we can see all of this from the forest plot. Although as I said earlier, we don't want to get into the habit of counting significant and non-significant papers, especially since we can pool the studies together.

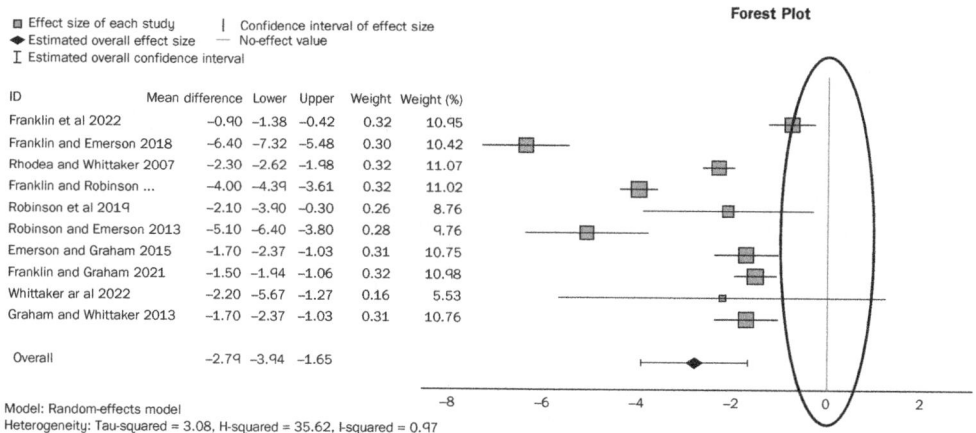

Figure 13.3 Example forest plot (with sample size removed to make the image bigger)

The black vertical line at 0 is the line of no effect. If a 95 per cent CI of an included paper crosses 0 (when looking at mean difference), then the results would be non-significant. The 'Overall' row provides our pooled statistics. So, for this example the pooled mean difference would be −2.79, 95 per cent CI (−3.94 to −1.65). The diamond is the pooled mean difference represented on the forest plot. When we have minus mean differences then this means the score in the comparison group was higher than the intervention group. If the values were positive, then the mean would have been higher in the intervention group compared to the comparison.

The 'Overall' row provides our pooled statistics, in the case, the pooled mean difference. When we pool all of our studies together and weigh these for sample size, this is the result we get. For me, this is what makes a meta-analysis really impressive: we've taken all the results from each of the individual studies and created this overall pooled statistic.

So, for this example the pooled mean difference would be –2.79, 95% CI (–3.94 to –1.65). We can also see this displayed in the forest plot by a diamond, which is the pooled mean difference represented on the forest plot.

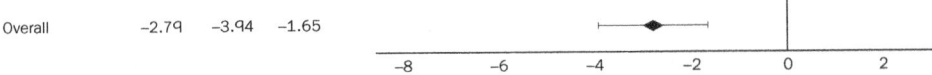

| Overall | –2.79 | –3.94 | –1.65 |

Figure 13.4 Overall pooled statisitc.

In this example meta-analysis, we can see that the pooled statistic is –2.79. This means that searching skill was higher in the comparison group, which was onsite learning. So based on these 10 studies, evidence would suggest that onsite learning resulted in higher searching skill scores compared to online learning (although, as I say, I've made this data up) and this is what the meta-analysis tells us. However, there is something else we need to think about when we report the results from a meta-analysis: the first is the pooled statistic and the second thing to report is how much heterogeneity there is. Well, what does heterogeneity mean?

Summary

- A forest plot provides us with a picture of our data.
- We can look at the forest plot to see trends in our data.
- The forest plot provides us with the statistic we are using (in this example mean difference) and 95 per cent CI for each of our included papers.
- The longer the line, the wider the 95 per cent CI, which is linked to the sample size. Larger sample sizes result in narrower 95 per cent CI.
- In our example we've looked at mean difference. When we get a minus mean difference it means the score in the intervention group was lower than in the comparison group.
- When we get a positive mean difference, it means the score was lower in the comparison group than in the intervention group.
- For our example a high score was better than a low score, so as we have a minus mean difference the score in the intervention group was lower than the comparison group. In other words, online learning resulted in a lower score than onsite learning.
- We can report the pooled statistic, but we also need to provide some indication of heterogeneity.

Heterogeneity (or between-study difference) and the statistics used to assess it

Before we discuss statistical heterogeneity it's important to remember that you can only combine studies that have the same PICOT/PEOT components. So, for example, we should not be combining studies using different interventions or different study designs. It's usually inappropriate to combine different populations as well, although as always this would depend on your research question. The studies must be similar in their PICOT/PEOT components.

When we discuss meta-analysis another really important point to consider is called heterogeneity; this refers to *how much variability there is between the included studies*. This is important because if there is a lot of variability between the studies and we don't report this then we're not giving readers all the information they need to make decisions.

Let's look at Figures 13.5 and 13.6. They both have very similar pooled statistics (−2.15 and −2.17 respectively). Now look at the distribution of the papers in the forest plot. In the first (Figure 13.5) you can see all the papers are reporting results which are quite similar. Now look at the second (Figure 13.6). You can see there is a lot of variation in the results reported between each of the included papers. What I mean by this is that in the first forest plot (Figure 13.5) the studies are all reporting similar findings. In the second example (Figure 13.6) they are more scattered. This means there is more between-study variability; put another way, there is more heterogeneity.

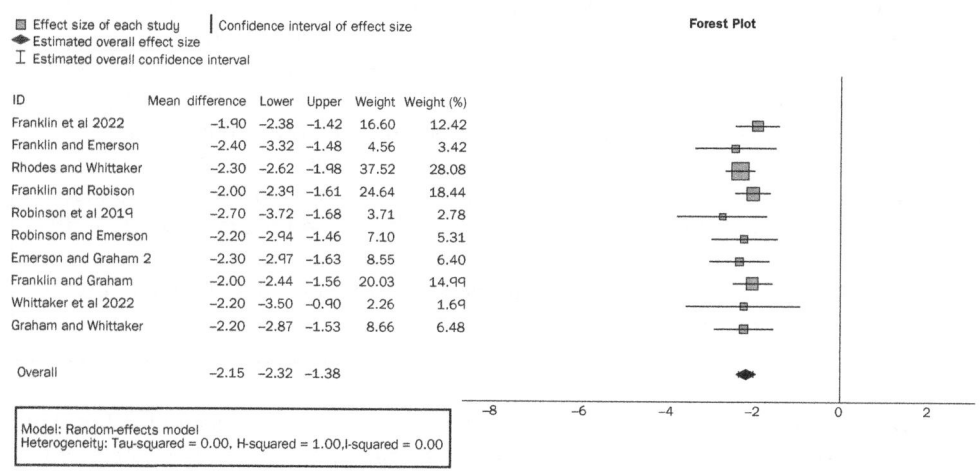

Figure 13.5 Example forest plot containing papers with quite similar results.

In the forest plot shown in Figure 13.5, the results from the included papers are all quite similar and in quite a neat column – there is less variability between the study findings.

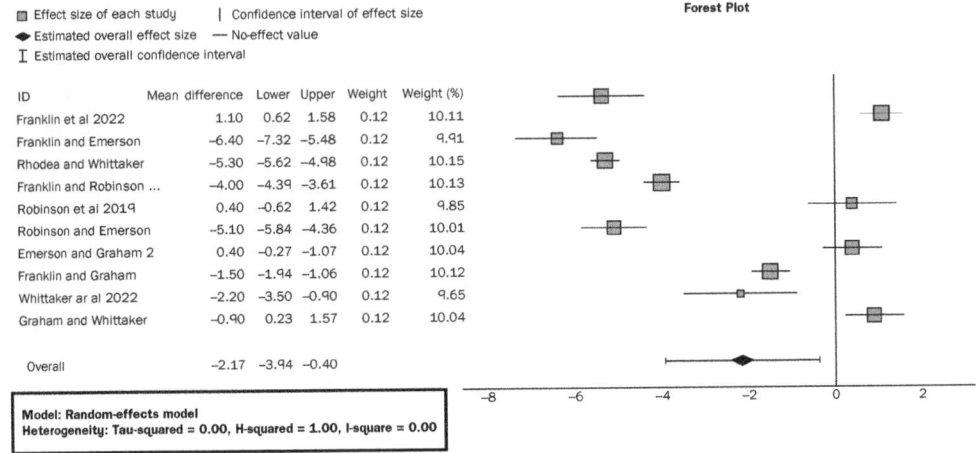

Figure 13.6 Example forest plot containing papers with more variability in their findings.

In the forest plot shown in Figure 13.6, the results from the included papers are more spread around – there is more variability in the study findings.

Case study 13.1

Now let's think about what this means in reality. Let's say you have the option of taking two medications. The research findings for medication A are summarized in Figure 13.5 and the results for medication B are summarized in Figure 13.6.

For medication A you can be reasonably confident that the results are fairly similar in all the papers. But for the second medication you have some papers that showed a really strong benefit in favour of the intervention while other papers favoured the control. I suspect most people would choose the medication that had findings that were similar to each other, as you can be more confident in the results (assuming the methodological quality of the papers is good). In the same way we report the SD alongside a mean in a primary study, we should also provide some indication of heterogeneity alongside the pooled statistic, otherwise our results might be misleading.

The outcomes of the meta-analyses in Figures 13.5 and 13.6 are very similar, but there is more heterogeneity (or variability in study findings) in Figure 13.6. We need to report the pooled statistic and provide some indication of heterogeneity.

I-squared

The most commonly used statistic to quantify heterogeneity is I-squared (I^2). If you look at the two forest plots in Figures 13.5 and 13.6, you can see it in the 'Heterogeneity' section in the bottom left-hand corner. This is provided as a value between 0 and 1 and we then report it as a percentage. So, 0.99 would be 99 per cent. Also see Figure 13.7.

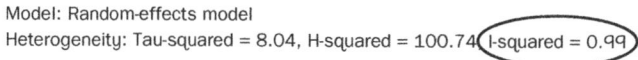

Model: Random-effects model
Heterogeneity: Tau-squared = 8.04, H-squared = 100.74, I-squared = 0.99

Figure 13.7 Example of outputs which show heterogeneity.

The Cochrane Handbook (Deeks et al. 2023) provides the following thresholds for I^2:

- 0 per cent to 40 per cent: might not be important.
- 30 per cent to 60 per cent: may represent moderate heterogeneity.
- 50 per cent to 90 per cent: may represent substantial heterogeneity.
- 75 per cent to 100 per cent: considerable heterogeneity.

Tau and 95 per cent Prediction interval

Tau is the statistic of between-study variability and is interpreted a bit like a standard deviation. In effect, if tau is large then there is a lot of between-study variability; if tau is small then there is less between-study variability. Tau is reported in the same units as the pooled statistic so we can see clearly how much variability there is in the units in which we're working.

The last point to note is that when reporting the results of a random-effects meta-analysis we should report the 95 per cent prediction interval (PI). We can interpret this in a similar way to a 95 per cent CI, in that the wider this interval the less precision there is around our pooled statistic. Now, for me this is the basics of interpreting a meta-analysis. For the second half of this chapter we'll talk through how to run a meta-analysis and do a little more theory along the way as well.

Summary

- Heterogeneity tells us about how much between-study variability there is between our included studies.
- It's essential that we provide information about statistical heterogeneity by reporting statistics such as I^2 and tau and, when using a random-effects meta-analysis, the 95 per cent PI.

Running a basic meta-analysis

The first things to consider when running your analysis are:

1   What do you want to know?
2   What data will you need to answer your research question?

When we do any data analysis, the approach we use should be driven by our research aims. You should therefore be really clear about what you want to find out before you begin analysing your data.

> **Task***:*
>
> Write your research aim out in a PICOT/PEOT format.
>
> What is your outcome? What is it specifically that you want to know about?
>
> Remember to try and maintain clarity of message in your work. The outcome in your question is what we need to analyse.

1. What data points are we comparing?

Often in clinical research we are using data from RCTs and we are comparing the effectiveness of a treatment or intervention compared to a control, comparison or placebo group. We will usually have at least four data points (if not more), so how do we choose what to use? As always, the best resource to support this question – and the one I would recommend – is the Cochrane Handbook (Higgins et al. 2023). However, I will summarize some of the choices we have available to us:

1   We use the post only data. With data from an RCT we can assume the groups are roughly equal at baseline and therefore we can use the post only data.

2   We use the change data (i.e., the change from baseline to post-test). However, unfortunately more often than not a lot of researchers don't report the change data – which as you start doing more meta-analyses you quickly realize is incredibly frustrating. Now, you can estimate the change data, but these are only estimates and it's quite an involved process so I would suggest, at this level, if we are using data from RCTs we stick with post only data.

> **Practical Tip**
>
> A meta-analysis compares two points, so this might be a comparison between a treatment group and a control group, or it might be pre and post data. Either way we can only compare two points.

2. Are the data in the correct format?

For us to run our meta-analysis we need the mean, standard deviation (SD) and the sample size for each group. However, sometimes authors will report the standard error (of the mean), abbreviated to SE or SEM. Now it's really important that we spot this, and we change the data to the required format – if we don't, it will mean our analysis is incorrect and we'll report an incorrect pooled statistic.

It's important to look over the papers carefully and see how they are reporting their data. If the paper stated Mean ± SD, then this is fine; we can input this straight into our analysis. However, if the paper states 'values are Mean ± SEM' or SE (or words to this effect), we need to convert this using the formula below, taken from the Cochrane Handbook (Higgins et al. 2023).

$$SD = SE \times \sqrt{N}$$

To convert the SE(M) to an SD we simply multiply the SE by the square root of the sample size for that group. So, if the SE was 8 and the sample size for that group is 5, we simply multiply 8 by the square root of 5 and we get an SD of 17.9. It's really important that we ensure that the data that we have inputted into our analysis are in the correct format.

3. Are there more than two groups?

Remember, we've said we can only compare two data points, so what do we do if we have more than two groups? For example, there might be one control group and two intervention groups. You might be tempted to say: 'Well, I'll include the paper twice, once for each of my intervention groups.' But you shouldn't do this, as we should only include each paper in our meta-analysis once. We shouldn't include the same paper multiple times.

Therefore, we have two options available to us:

1   We use only one of the intervention groups and compare those data against the comparison group only; we ignore the other intervention group.

2   We can combine the two intervention groups together. However, this process can be a little complicated and therefore I'm not going to describe it in this chapter. As with everything related to meta-analysis (and systematic reviews), how to do this is detailed in the Cochrane Handbook (Higgins et al. 2023). We just need to ensure, if we are combining groups, that these groups are similar enough to be combined.

The important thing to remember is that you can't include the same paper more than once in the same analysis.

4. What if the outcome I am using has been measured by multiple different measurement tools across my included papers?

When we are using patient-reported outcomes, we often use measurement tools to capture this data. However, it's very common for there to be multiple scales that are all measuring the same underlying construct.

For example, let's say we want to measure fatigue in a particular population. The included papers may have used the Fatigue Severity Scale (FSS) or the Chalder Fatigue Scale (CFS). If using the CFS we might use the 14-item version, or we might use the 11-item version. Here we have three different measurement tools, but they're all measuring the same underlying construct (in this example, fatigue). So, how do we meta-analyse these different measurement scales? There are two ways in which we can deal with this.

1. The easiest way to deal with this is to convert these measurements into a common metric, and a useful common metric is percentages. We can convert each of these scores to a percentage and then we can meta-analyse these percentage scores. The good thing about percentages is that most people understand percentages and they make sense to people, so it's easier to explain our findings.

2. The other option is to use standardized mean difference (SMD). SPSS can calculate this for you. It basically converts the scores into an effect size, such as Cohen's d, and then meta-analyses these scores. This is useful as the software does the conversion for you; however, I often find that not everyone understands Cohen's d in the same way they do percentages.

Practical Tips

- We need to ensure we have the appropriate data to input into our meta-analysis – if the data aren't in the correct format, then we either exclude them from the analysis or we convert the data.
- We should document each stage to ensure our work can be replicated.
- If the data aren't in the correct format, it can be a good idea to contact authors directly and ask for the data. If you contact authors, you should report whom you contacted and how this impacted your analysis (i.e., you used data directly from the author).

Inputting the data

OK, so hopefully we've successfully extracted the correct data and we've made the relevant conversions to allow us to run the meta-analysis. Let's look at how we input some data into SPSS and then how to run a random-effects meta-analysis. I've included a dataset in Figure 13.8 that you can practise with. It is the same dataset that I'll be using in these examples.

Study	Intervention			Control		
	Sample	Mean	SD	Sample	Mean	SD
Study 1	20	6.9	3.20	20	5.20	2.60
Study 2	64	5.7	3.80	52	3.30	3.30
Study 3	108	5.6	4.00	110	3.00	1.50
Study 4	205	6.5	3.50	205	4.40	2.40
Study 5	152	8.3	3.20	152	6.90	1.80
Study 6	320	6.2	2.80	320	3.80	2.50
Study 7	167	6.5	2.70	167	4.50	3.50
Study 8	254	6.2	2.20	254	3.80	3.20
Study 9	100	8.3	3.40	100	5.50	5.10
Study 10	84	5.6	5.20	84	4.30	2.30

Figure 13.8 Example dataset for practice meta-analysis.

Firstly, when you first load an SPSS spreadsheet, in the 'Variable View' create the rows to allow you to input the data.

If you're not familiar with SPSS, you just need to label your variables in the 'Variable View' and then you can input the data in the 'Data View'. You can toggle between these two (see Figure 13.9) using the icons in the bottom left of the spreadsheet. To name our variables we need to go to the Variable View.

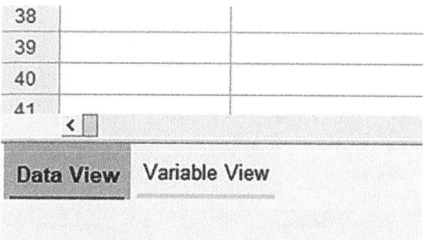

Figure 13.9 Data View and Variable View in SPSS.

We then need to create the variables for the analysis. In this case we'll need Study ID, the sample size, mean and SD for the intervention and the sample size, and the mean and SD for the comparison group. Figure 13.10 provides an example of how you can label your variables in the Variable View section. When you label your variables, don't leave any spaces between words. So Study ID needs to be 'StudyID'.

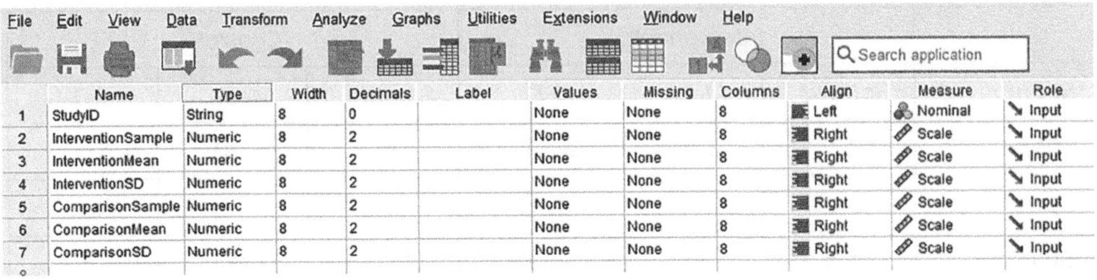

	Name	Type	Width	Decimals	Label	Values	Missing	Columns	Align	Measure	Role
1	StudyID	String	8	0		None	None	8	Left	Nominal	Input
2	InterventionSample	Numeric	8	2		None	None	8	Right	Scale	Input
3	InterventionMean	Numeric	8	2		None	None	8	Right	Scale	Input
4	InterventionSD	Numeric	8	2		None	None	8	Right	Scale	Input
5	ComparisonSample	Numeric	8	2		None	None	8	Right	Scale	Input
6	ComparisonMean	Numeric	8	2		None	None	8	Right	Scale	Input
7	ComparisonSD	Numeric	8	2		None	None	8	Right	Scale	Input

Figure 13.10 Creating the variables in the Variable View in SPSS.

We then need to toggle to the Data View by pressing on the icon in the bottom left corner. We can then copy and paste our data from Figure 13.8 directly into our spreadsheet, as shown in Figure 13.11.

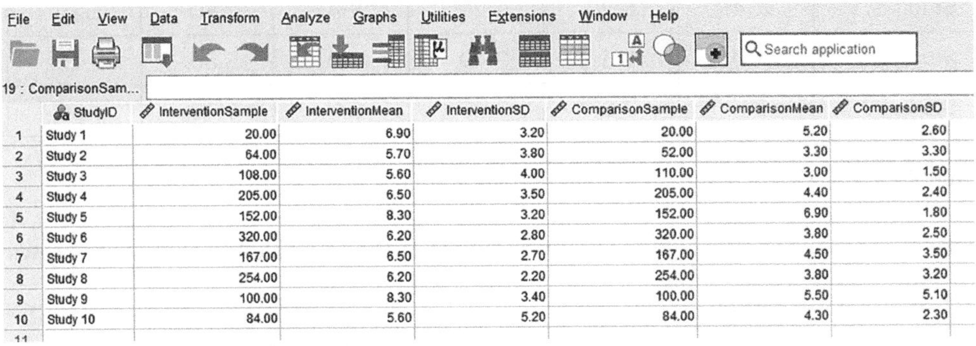

	StudyID	InterventionSample	InterventionMean	InterventionSD	ComparisonSample	ComparisonMean	ComparisonSD
1	Study 1	20.00	6.90	3.20	20.00	5.20	2.60
2	Study 2	64.00	5.70	3.80	52.00	3.30	3.30
3	Study 3	108.00	5.60	4.00	110.00	3.00	1.50
4	Study 4	205.00	6.50	3.50	205.00	4.40	2.40
5	Study 5	152.00	8.30	3.20	152.00	6.90	1.80
6	Study 6	320.00	6.20	2.80	320.00	3.80	2.50
7	Study 7	167.00	6.50	2.70	167.00	4.50	3.50
8	Study 8	254.00	6.20	2.20	254.00	3.80	3.20
9	Study 9	100.00	8.30	3.40	100.00	5.50	5.10
10	Study 10	84.00	5.60	5.20	84.00	4.30	2.30

Figure 13.11 Adding the data to the Data View in SPSS.

For this example, we're going to run a meta-analysis on the mean difference between the two groups. To do this we need to go to 'Analyze', then 'Meta-Analysis', 'Continuous Outcomes' and then 'Raw Data', as shown in Figure 13.12.

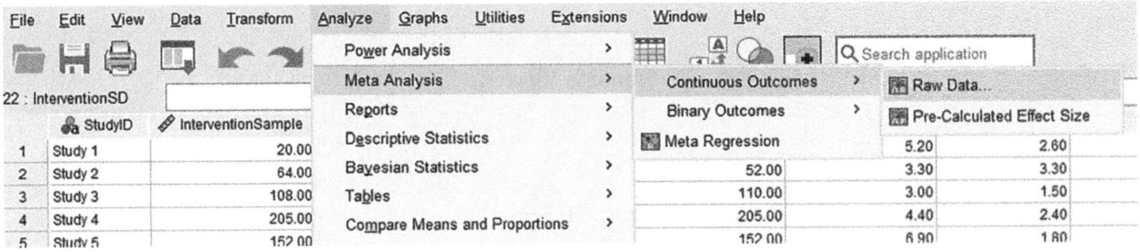

Figure 13.12 How to select the meta-analysis function in SPSS.

When we are in the dialogue box for the meta-analysis, we just need to input the correct variable into the appropriate box; then, for the Effect Size, change this to 'Unstandardized Mean Difference'. This means that we will report the pooled statistic as the mean difference, and we aren't going to be reporting a standardized mean difference. How this should look can be seen in Figure 13.13.

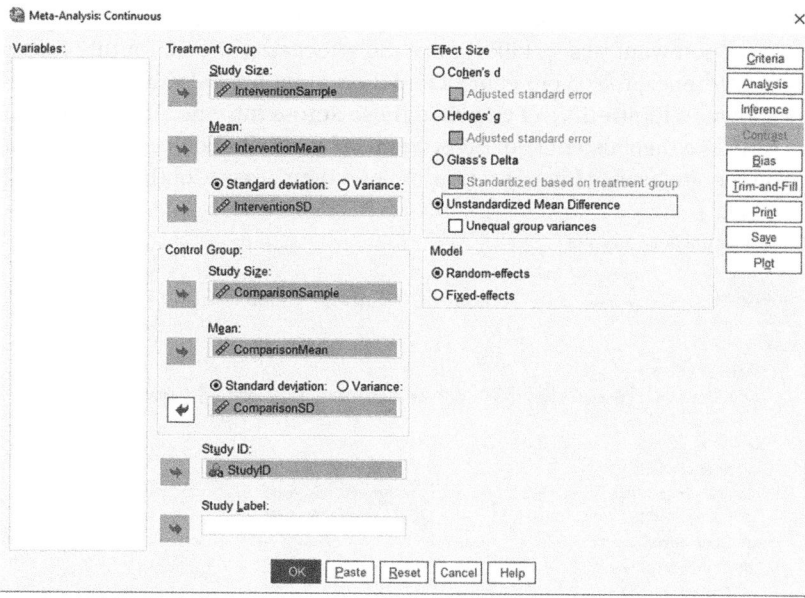

Figure 13.13 Moving the variables into the correct box in SPSS.

Select 'Print' and 'Heterogeneity measures' and select 'Prediction interval under random-effects model', as shown in Figure 13.14. This will provide us with 95 per cent PI so we can report this in our findings.

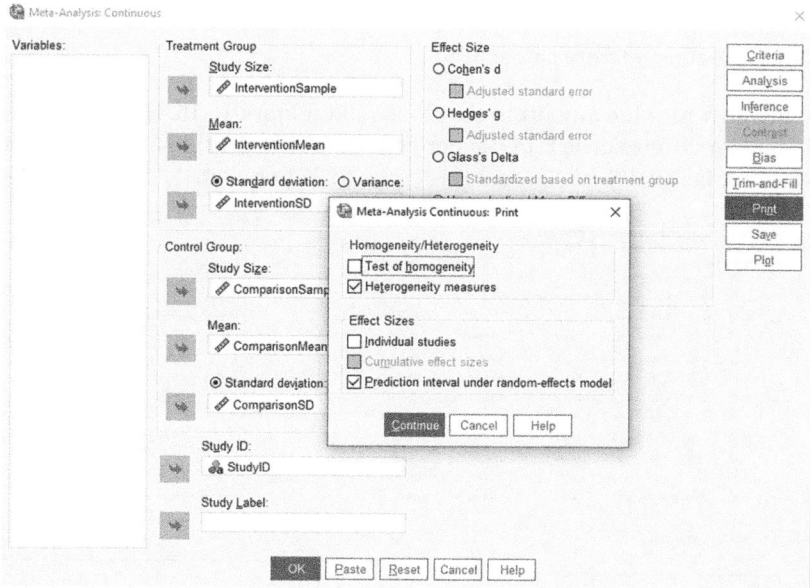

Figure 13.14 Selecting prediction interval in SPSS.

Then, in 'Plot', we'll create our forest plot. Click on 'Plot'. In this section, set this to display the information you want to see. I like to see the effect size, which, for this example, will be the mean difference, the 95 per cent CI and the weighting. I also like to see the sample size, so as shown in Figure 13.15 I've pulled these across into the 'Additional Column(s)' section as well. I've then also ticked 'Heterogeneity' in the 'Annotations' section and 'Null effect size' in the 'Reference Lines' section. We can then press 'Continue' and 'OK'.

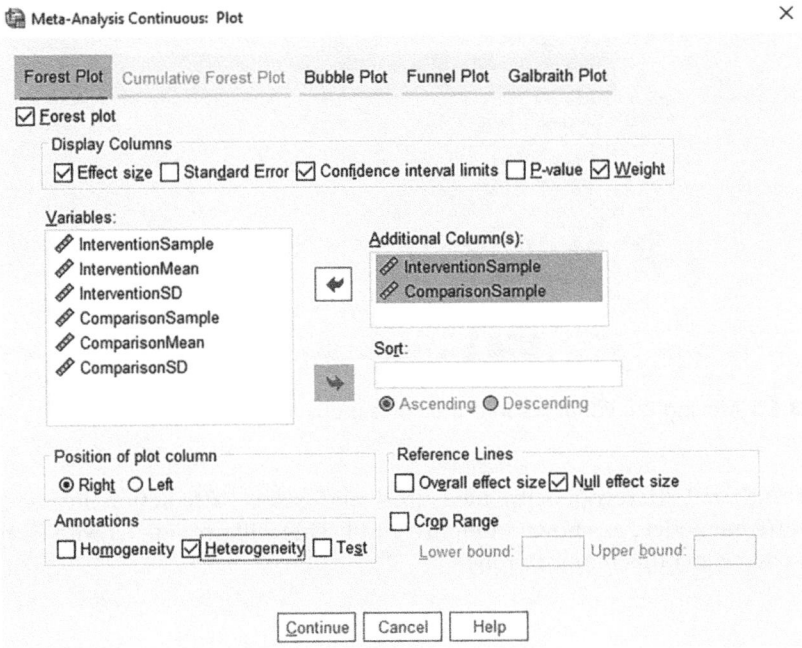

Figure 13.15 Creating a forest plot in SPSS.

SPSS should now provide an output that looks like Figure 13.16. Here we can see that the pooled mean difference is 2.14 (95 per cent CI 1.85 to 2.44), tau is 0.28 (square root of Tau-squared, i.e. $\sqrt{0.08} = 0.28$) and I^2 is equal to 37 per cent.

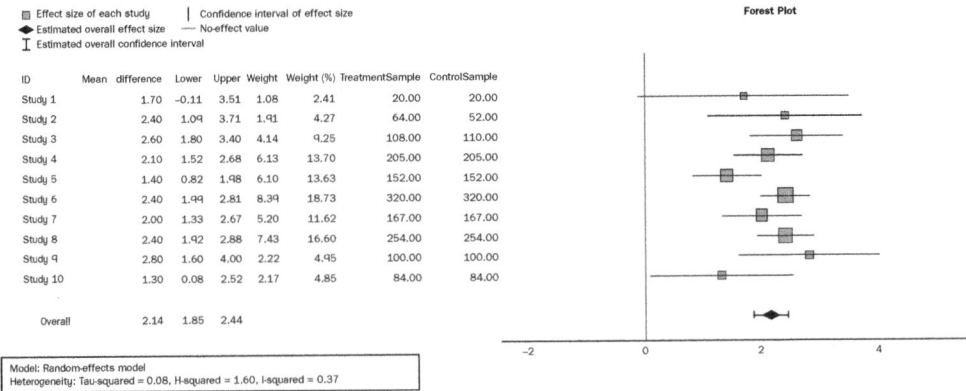

Figure 13.16 An example forest plot in SPSS.

We also get the output shown in Figure 13.17, which provides us with the 95 per cent PI.

Effect Size Estimates

	Effect Size	Std. Error	Z	Sig. (2-tailed)	95% Confidence Interval Lower	Upper	95% Prediction Interval[a] Lower	Upper
Overall	2.144	.1494	14.350	<.001	1.851	2.437	1.424	2.864

a. Based on t-distribution.

Figure 13.17 Prediction interval for an example meta-analysis in SPSS.

We can now report everything we need for this example analysis. We can report the pooled mean difference, tau and I^2 and the 95 per cent PI.

Reporting the output from the meta-analysis

When we report the meta-analysis, it is a good idea to present the forest plot and then report the key information alongside this. These include the pooled statistic and the 95 per cent CI, alongside the measures of heterogeneity and the 95 per cent PI (if you have conducted a random-effects meta-analysis).

To run your meta-analysis, you need to have the mean, SD and sample size. You can use the template in Table 13.2 to extract the correct data for your own review. Table 13.2 also provides an example of how data can be inputted into the analysis.

Table 13.2 Template for extracting the appropriate data for a meta-analysis

	Intervention			Control		
Study	Sample size	Mean	SD	Sample size	Mean	SD

🔑 Key points

- We can only run a meta-analysis if the studies have very similar PICOT/PEOT components.
- We need to ensure our data are in the appropriate format before we run the analysis.
- It's important that we provide information about statistical heterogeneity, as this is a really important aspect of how we interpret our findings.
- When we report the findings of a random-effects meta-analysis we should include the pooled statistic, the measures of heterogeneity and the 95 per cent PI.

Summary

- A meta-analysis is a way of synthesizing the results from multiple papers to create a new overall pooled statistic.
- It's important to make sure we provide information about the statistical heterogeneity as well as the overall results.
- A forest plot is an effective way to show our findings and the variation in the individual study findings.

References

Campbell, M., McKenzie, J.E., Sowden, A., et al. (2020) Synthesis without meta-analysis (SWiM) in systematic reviews: Reporting guideline. *British Medical Journal* 368: l6890.

Deeks, J.J., Higgins, J.P.T. and Altman, D.G. (2023) Chapter 10: Analysing data and undertaking meta-analyses. In J.P.T. Higgins, J. Thomas, J. Chandler et al. (eds). *Cochrane Handbook for Systematic Reviews of Interventions*, version 6.4 (updated August 2023). Available at www.training.cochrane.org/handbook (accessed 24 November 2023)

Higgins, J.P.T., Thomas, J., Chandler, J. et al. (eds) (2023) *Cochrane Handbook for Systematic Reviews of Interventions*, version 6.4 (updated August 2023). Available at www.training.cochrane.org/handbook (accessed 24 November 2023).

Popay, J., Roberts, H., Sowden, A. et al. (2006) Guidance on the conduct of narrative synthesis in systematic reviews: A product from the ESRC methods programme. Version 1(1), p.b92. https://doi.org/10.13140/2.1.1018.4643.

Thomas, J. and Harden, A. (2008) Methods for the thematic synthesis of qualitative research in systematic reviews. *BMC Medical Research Methodology* 8 (1): 1–10.

Index

Page numbers in italics are figures; with 't' are tables; in bold are boxes.

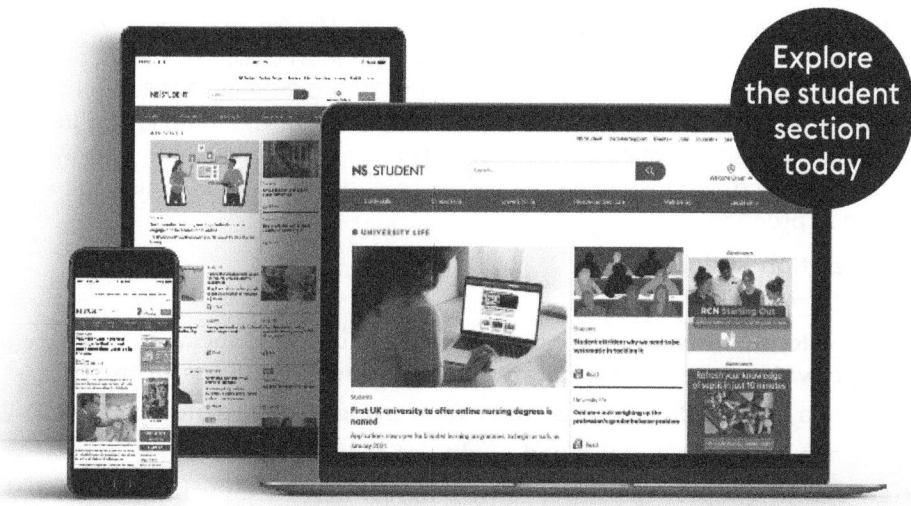
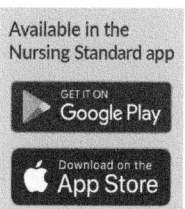

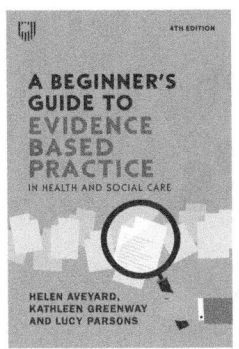

A Beginner's Guide to Evidence-Based Practice in Health and Social Care

Helen Aveyard, Kathleen Greenway, Lucy Parsons

4th edition

ISBN: 9780335251964 (Paperback)
eISBN: 9780335251971

2023

A Beginner's Guide to Evidence-Based Practice in Health and Social Care, 4th edition is the book for anyone who has ever wondered what evidence-based practice is, or how to relate it to practice or use it in academic work. Thoroughly revised with two new co-authors this brand new edition uses simple and jargon-free language to help those new to the topic. It provides an accessible step-by-step guide to what we mean by evidence in practice and how to apply this concept to learning and practice.

This new edition features:

- **New explanations with examples from both health and social care practice, using a wide range of research that is also relevant outside of the UK**
- **Coverage of new discourse on the use of evidence generated by COVID-19**
- **Coverage on the role, need and quality of rapid reviews**
- **New end-of-chapter questions to help assess how much you have learned**

This book provides an inter-professional approach and is key reading for both students and professionals who need to search for, appraise and apply evidence across nursing, allied health care or social care.

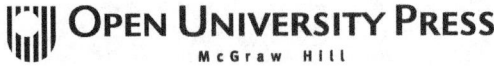
OPEN UNIVERSITY PRESS
McGraw Hill

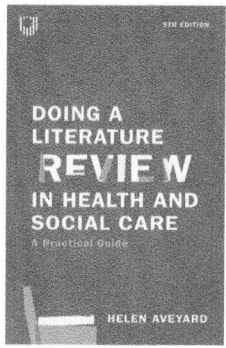

Doing a Literature Review in Health and Social Care:
A Practical Guide

Helen Aveyard

5th edition

ISBN: 9780335251940 (Paperback)
eISBN: 9780335251957

2023

This best-selling book, now in its fifth edition, is a step-by-step guide to doing a literature review for students in all areas of health and social care. It is essential reading for all those doing their undergraduate dissertation or any study that involves doing a literature review.

The new edition maintains its signature 'can do' approach and provides a practical guide to doing a literature review from start to finish. This book includes:

- **A broad and updated range of real life examples of how to overcome challenges in the process**
- **Tips on how to get your question right**
- **Updated guidance on following a clear search strategy for relevant literature using the appropriate technology**
- **Brand new and accessible chapter summaries**
- **An expanded guide for the application of critical appraisal tools**
- **An increased emphasis on presenting your findings or using them in practice**

Doing a Literature Review in Health and Social Care is vital reading for anyone new to reviewing and presenting evidence in a review

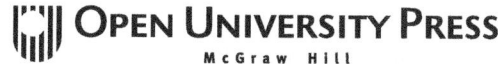

OPEN UNIVERSITY PRESS
McGraw Hill

www.mheducation.co.uk

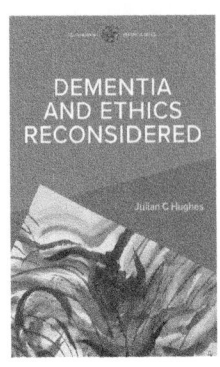

Dementia and Ethics Reconsidered

Julian Hughes

ISBN: 9780335251001 (Paperback)
eISBN: 9780335251018

2023

Ethical issues are involved in every decision that is made in connection with someone living with dementia – from decisions about care and treatment to decisions about research and funding.

This book encourages the reader to reconsider ethics in dementia care with the use of 'patterns of practice', an innovative idea developed by the author. The book highlights the importance of understanding the person's narrative, of good communication, high quality care, and expert interpretation of the meaning of situations for people living with dementia. This book:

- Reviews ethical theories and approaches in connection with dementia care
- Considers issues such as stigma, quality of life, personhood and citizenship in relation to dementia
- Looks at issues relevant to research ethics
- Presents case vignettes to highlight a complete spectrum of ethical issues that arise in dementia care
- Is accessibly written for multiple audiences – from people living with dementia to practitioners

Dementia and Ethics Reconsidered is a comprehensive account of thought and practice in relation to ethical issues that arise in the context of dementia care, which seeks to show how ethical thinking can be put into practice and prove relevant to day-to-day experience.

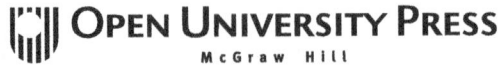

www.mheducation.co.uk